The

ULCERATIVE COLITIS

COOKBOOK

1600+

DAYS OF QUICK & EASY RECIPES TO QUICKLY IMPROVE GUT HEALTH AND A 28-DAY MEAL
PLAN TO IMPROVE YOUR WELL-BEING

Maxwell Baers

TABLE OF CONTENTS

INTRODUCTION

Ulcerative Colitis is a dangerous disease, with approximately 500,000 new cases reported annually. In America, at least five million are affected by this disease. There are different types of ulcer disease, but peptic ulcer disease is most common in people born in the mid-20th century. Ulcer illness primarily affects the elderly, with a peak incidence between the ages of 55 and 65. Usually, duodenal ulcers are more common in men than in women, and 35% of gastric ulcer patients will experience complications. Despite low mortality rates, peptic ulcer disease's high incidence, pain, suffering, and costs remain high.

This cookbook was created to assist newly diagnosed ulcer patients. Choosing safe food to eat when you have an ulcer disease for the first time can be difficult. This cookbook will be highly beneficial; utilize it wisely if you want to thrive despite your situation. Thanks to a 28-day meal plan and 120 delectable, healthful dishes, you can prepare and eat meals with pride.

Different studies suggest certain dietary adjustments may help prevent and heal stomach ulcers. Anyone who has an ulcer should follow an ulcer diet. An ulcer diet is designed to alleviate the discomfort produced by a peptic/stomach ulcer, a painful wound on the stomach, esophagus, and small intestine. It may also help cure gastritis or stomach inflammation. Although your doctor is more likely to treat your ulcer with medication than food alone, adding a diet to your treatment plan may help you feel better faster and avoid another ulcer.

Following an ulcer diet with other treatment recommendations may be beneficial because it can alleviate nutritional deficiencies contributing to your symptoms while providing protein and other healing elements. Avoid foods that irritate your stomach or small intestine, as this will aid in the control of Crohn's disease, bacterial infections, and celiac disease, which may be causing your ulcer.

CHAPTER 1:
What is Ulcerative Colitis?

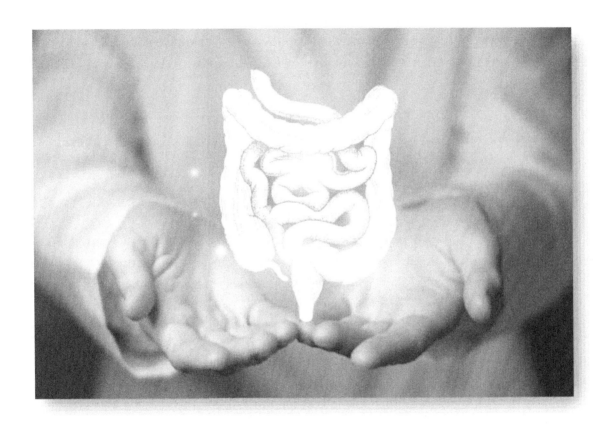

Ulcerative Colitis is a condition caused by an overactive immune system that begins to attack your own body. It all starts when your colon lining becomes inflamed. If this is not addressed, the inflammation causes small open ulcers and sores on the lining of your colon.

In some people, ulcerative colitis is a protracted process that begins with inflammation. Unfortunately, we have become accustomed to seeking a quick remedy rather than delving deeper to determine the root cause of an issue. In this situation, many of us turn to over-the-counter medicine to provide instant relief from the abdominal pain we are experiencing. This band-aid technique may provide short relief, but the pain and discomfort linger, and we may take additional medications until the pain and discomfort become severe enough that we seek medical assistance.

Unfortunately, the condition has already progressed to the point that open ulcers and sores in the colon lining exist. After being diagnosed with ulcerative colitis, you will experience flare-ups and remissions in which the painful symptoms will diminish. The goal is to stay in remission for as long as possible, which can range from weeks to years, depending on the severity of your disease and the therapies you've taken.

According to research, the following people are predisposed to ulcerative colitis:

- People with a relative, either a parent, child or brother/sister, suffer from any form of Inflammatory Bowel Disease.
- People between the ages of mid-teenage, that is, 15 to 30 years. It's crucial to remember that Ulcerative colitis can strike at any age. It's just that it is most common between 15–30-year-old.
- People of Jewish descent. Though the reason is unsure, they seem to have more cases of ulcerative colitis.

Causes of Ulcerative Colitis

When it comes to ulcerative colitis, doctors and medical researchers have not pinpointed the exact cause of the disease. However, they think the following factors contribute to one having ulcerative colitis.

An Excessive Immune Function

Your immune system's principal duty is to keep your body safe by fighting off dangerous and possibly harmful germs that attack it. When you are harmed, your immune system also assists you in healing.

However, your immune system can occasionally go astray and begin confusing food and healthy microorganisms in your gut for hazardous ones. In this case, the immune system launches an attack through inflammation to isolate the afflicted or infected area so that the problem may be addressed as quickly as possible and your body can return to top condition.

Chronic inflammation occurs when inflammation repeatedly occurs, especially when there is no real threat. You will have abdominal pain if you have ulcerative colitis since your colon is always inflamed. If not treated, this can result in ulcers and even rips, both of which can be harmful.

Genetics

Suppose you have a family history of ulcerative colitis or another type of Irritable Bowel Disease (IBD). In that case, you are at a greater risk of acquiring ulcerative colitis or another type of IBD. However, it is crucial to note that most ulcerative colitis patients do not have a family history of the condition. As a result, doctors and researchers focus on establishing the disease's environmental source.

Surroundings

Ulcerative colitis may be connected to pollution and other environmental variables. For example, smoking has been linked to an increased risk of developing IBD. The number of persons presenting with ulcerative colitis is expanding at an alarming rate in an increasingly hazardous world.

Microbiomes of the Gut

Your stomach is home to bacteria, viruses, and fungi. Some are healthy and aid digestion, while others are harmful and can cause illness. The good microbiome should constantly outnumber the harmful microbiome to remain healthy. According to studies, people with ulcerative colitis and IBD have distinct microbiomes from those without the disease.

Even though everyone has a unique collection of microbiomes, researchers are trying to figure out why people with ulcerative colitis and other irritable bowel diseases have such significantly different microbiomes and what this means for treatment.

Symptoms Of Ulcerative Colitis

These symptoms might vary based on the inflammation's degree and location. Possible signs and symptoms include:

- Fever
- Urgency to defecate
- Inability to defecate despite urgency
- Rectal pain
- Abdominal pain and cramping
- Fatigue
- Diarrhea, often with blood or pus
- In children, failure to grow
- Rectal bleeding
- Weight loss

Most individuals with ulcerative colitis exhibit mild to moderate symptoms. The progression of ulcerative colitis might vary, with some patients experiencing lengthy remissions.

CHAPTER 2:
Foods To Avoid And Foods To Eat

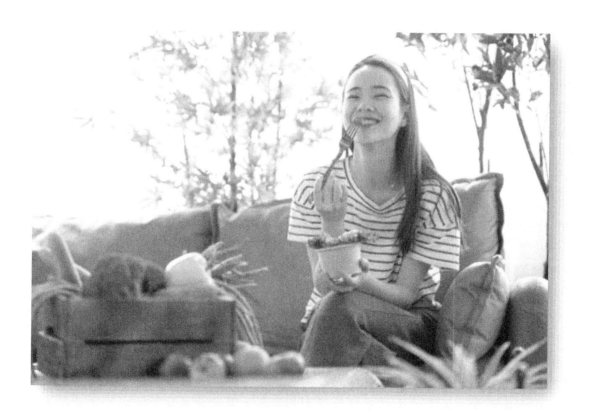

Unlike other diet programs, a low-residue diet offers a wide variety of foods that can be consumed. This chapter will detail foods from various food groups that should be included and avoided.

Bread and Starches

The following is a list of allowed foods and foods to avoid for the Bread and Starches food group.

Allowed Foods

- White bread

- Muffins
- Rolls
- Biscuits
- Crackers
- Light rye bread (seedless)
- Pancakes
- Waffles
- Corn flakes
- Rice Krispies
- Puffed rice
- White potatoes
- Sweet potatoes (without skin)
- White rice
- Refined Pasta
- Refined cooked cereals

Foods To Avoid

- Wholemeal bread and flour
- Granary bread and flour
- Wholemeal pasta
- Quinoa
- Pearl barley
- Brown rice
- All cereals that contain whole wheat
- Muesli
- Porridge

Note: Products made with coconut, nuts, bran, seeds, or dried fruits are extremely high in fiber and leave a great amount of residue and hence are not recommended in this diet.

Meat and Protein

The following is a list of allowed foods and foods to avoid for Meat and Protein.

Allowed Foods

- Ground, tender, or well-cooked lean meats
- Poultry
- Tofu
- Fish

- Eggs
- Creamy peanut butter

Foods To Avoid

- Tough and gristly meat
- Skin and bones of fish

Vegetables

The following is a list of the allowed and must-be-avoided foods in the Vegetables food group.

Allowed Foods

- Cucumber
- Green pepper
- Romaine
- Tomatoes
- Onions
- Zucchini
- Carrots

Foods To Avoid

- Legumes
- Raw high-fiber vegetables
- Split peas
- Lentils
- Peas
- Sweet corn
- All seeds
- All pips
- All tough skins
- Potato skins
- Baked beans
- Lima beans
- Green peas
- Broccoli
- Parsnips
- Juices with pulp or bits

Note: Other vegetables are allowed except the ones seen in the list above.

Fruits

The following is a list of allowed foods and foods to avoid for the Fruits food group.

Allowed Foods

- Apricot
- Peach
- Plum
- Honeydew
- Nectarine
- Papaya
- Banana
- Cantaloupe
- Watermelon
- All juices without pulp and strained

Foods To Avoid

- All dried fruits and fruits with seeds

Note: All fruits except those not recommended or those with seeds or skins are allowed.

CHAPTER 3:
Breakfast

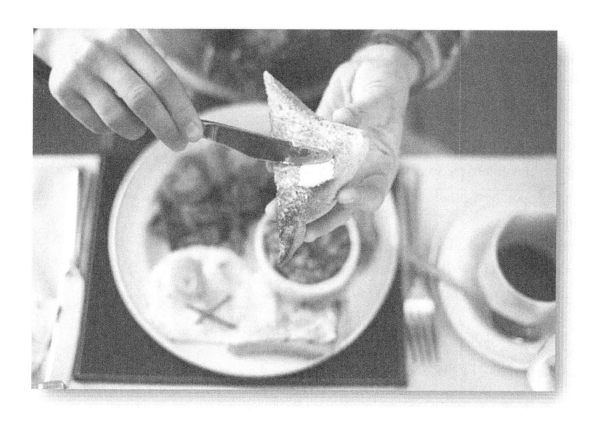

1. Soup of Butternut Squash

Preparation Time: 10 minutes

Cooking Time: 20 minutes

Servings: 6

Ingredients:

- 6 c. chicken stock
- 1 medium onion
- ½ c. Greek yogurt
- ½ tsp. nutmeg
- 2 tbsps. olive oil
- Salt and black pepper
- 1 3-lb. butternut squash

Directions:

1. Cut the squash into pieces that are 1 inch in size.
2. In a large pot, heat either olive oil or butter. Sauté the onion for about 8 minutes or until it becomes translucent.
3. Combine the squash and stock.
4. Mix the ingredients in the saucepan using an immersion (hand-held) blender until fully smooth.
5. Before transferring it to a regular blender, allow the soup to cool slightly.
6. Season with salt, pepper, and salt again after adding the nutmeg.
7. Garnish with a dollop of Greek yogurt if preferred.

Nutrition: Calories: 100, Fat: 3g, Sodium: 250 mg, Protein: 4 g, Carbs: 15 g

2. Sweet Potato Ginger Pancakes

Preparation Time: 10 minutes

Cooking Time: 25 minutes

Servings: 18 pancakes

Ingredients:

- 2 tsp. ginger
- Black pepper
- ¼ tsp. kosher salt
- ¼ c. almond flour
- 1 lb. sweet potatoes
- Cooking spray
- ¼ tsp. baking powder
- ¼ c. egg
- 1 medium onion

Directions:

1. Grate the potato and onion in a food processor fitted with a grating blade or with a handheld grater.
2. Place the mixture in a bowl. Mix in the ginger, egg substitute, flour, bicarbonate soda, salt, and pepper until well combined.
3. Spray a non-stick skillet with non-stick spray and heat it over low to medium heat.
4. Place ¼ cup of the potato mixture on the heated grill and flatten each pancake with the spatula's back side.
5. Cook the pancakes on each side for 6 to 8 minutes, flipping once the bottoms have turned golden brown.
6. Spray the pancakes with cooking spray before rotating them to keep them from sticking. Remove from the pan when both sides are toasted and slightly crunchy.
7. You can serve it immediately or reheat it in the microwave if necessary.

Nutrition: Calories: 110, Fat: 0 g, Sodium: 65 mg, Protein: 3 g, Carbs: 25

3. Apple and Banana Pancakes

Preparation Time: 10 minutes

Cooking Time: 15 minutes

Servings: 4

Ingredients:

- 5 medium chicken eggs
- 1 apple
- Honey
- 3 bananas
- 1 tbsp. coconut oil

Directions:

1. Peel the bananas before mashing them with a fork in a mixing basin.
2. After that, remove the core from the apple and combine it with the banana mixture.
3. Into the mixing bowl, break the eggs and then combine everything.
4. Begin by heating a frying pan (or two if you want to cook them faster), then add a little coconut oil to each pan as it heats.
5. Fill the pan with the mixture by dropping it in with a spoon. Each pan should be able to hold 3 to 4 pancakes. Spread the back of a spoon over each pancake and flatten it to make thin, circular pancakes.
6. Before removing the pancakes from the stove, wait until they are golden brown on one side, then turn them with a spatula. Cook for an additional minute after turning or until the opposite side is similarly golden brown.
7. Once done, remove it from the pan and cook the remaining ingredients in the same manner. After removing the pancakes from the skillet, arrange them on a dish to keep them warm.
8. Serve with honey (or anything else that tickles your fancy!) or on their own if you're trying to avoid sugars.

Nutrition: Calories: 60, Proteins: 1 g, Carbs: 13 g, Fat: 1 g

4. Lemon Bars

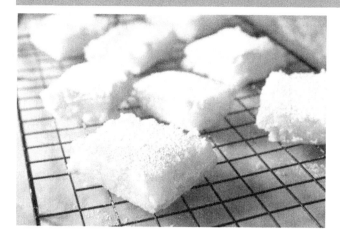

Preparation Time: 1 hour

Cooking Time: 25 minutes

Servings: 16

Ingredients:

For the Crust:

- ½ c. Coconut oil
- 2 Tbsp. sugar
- Pinch of salt
- 1 c. Coconut flour

For the Topping:

- 4 Eggs
- 2 tsp. Lemon zest
- ¾ c. Fresh lemon juice (about 6 large juicy lemons)
- ½ c. Sugar
- 1 ½ tsp. Coconut flour

Directions:

1. Apply coconut oil to an 8x8-inch baking sheet and preheat the oven to 350F. Set aside.
2. Combine the sugar, coconut oil, and a dash of salt in a large mixing bowl. When a dough starts to form, add the coconut flour and stir.
3. The dough should be uniformly spread throughout the prepared pan after about 10 minutes of baking. After cooking, allow to cool for 30 minutes.

4. Reduce the oven's heat setting to 325F. In a large mixing bowl, carefully whisk the eggs and lemon zest together when the crust has cooled.

5. In a separate bowl, gently heat the lemon juice. Mix thoroughly after adding the sugar. Stir the coconut flour into the lemon juice mixture, half a teaspoon at a time, until fully blended.

6. Whisk continually as you add the lemon juice mixture to the egg mixture to ensure even dispersion.

7. Spread the topping on top of the chilled crust. Bake for 20–22 minutes or until the topping is golden brown. Allow to cool completely at room temperature. After that, cover and place in the refrigerator for at least 6 hours, ideally overnight.

8. Using a sharp knife, cut the bars into squares.

Nutrition: Calories: 106, Proteins: 2.5 g, Carbs: 4.7 g, Fat: 8.9 g

5. Bacon-Wrapped Chicken, Pineapple, Roasted Veggies

Preparation Time: 15 minutes

Cooking Time: 30 minutes

Servings: 2

Ingredients:

- 1 large carrot
- 2 chicken breasts
- 2 tbsps. Coconut oil
- 1 medium sweet potato
- 4 bacon rashers
- 2 pineapples rings
- 1 large parsnip

Directions:

1. Preheat the oven to 200°C.
2. Make batons from the vegetables and remove the skins if you can't bear eating them. After that, lay the vegetables on a baking sheet and sprinkle them with coconut oil. If you dislike the flavor of coconut oil, you can substitute olive oil. Cook for 30 to 40 minutes in the oven.
3. Remove the saucepan from the oven and constantly swirl it to ensure that the vegetables are equally coated in the melted coconut oil. They should be golden in color and quite soft after cooking.'
4. Place a pineapple bell on top of each chicken breast, then wrap it with 2 strips of bacon, tying the ends beneath the chicken.
5. After about 10-15 minutes, transfer the vegetables to a second baking tray and set them in the oven.
6. After around 20-30 minutes in the oven, check to see if the chicken is ready to eat. When a knife is placed into the core of a perfectly cooked chicken, the juices should be clear. If you are doubtful, chop the chicken breast to inspect it. Cooking time can be influenced by various factors, including the chicken breast size and the oven used to prepare it. If the interior is still pink or crimson, wait 5 minutes before checking it again.
7. After cooking, remove the chicken and vegetables from the oven and serve.

Nutrition: Calories: 515, Proteins: 37 g, Carbs: 24 g, Fat: 22 g

6. Orange and Honey Duck

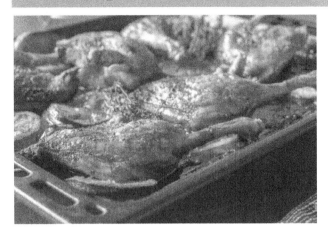

Preparation Time: 20 minutes

Cooking Time: 35 minutes

Servings: 2

Ingredients:

- 3 tbsps. Soy sauce
- 3 tbsps. Honey
- 2 duck breasts
- 1 orange juice and rind

Directions:

1. Preheat the oven to 200°C.
2. Combine the orange juice, rind, tamari, and honey on a plate. Next, add roasted duck breasts and coat them in the sauce before serving. Allow marinating for 15 minutes.
3. Once done, remove the breasts from the sauce, set them in an oven-safe dish, and bake for 10 to 15 minutes.
4. Set aside some of the sauce for later. Remove the duck from the oven and wrap it tightly in aluminum foil. Wait 5 minutes before proceeding.
5. Place the sauce in a small saucepan and let it come to a boil over high heat.
6. For a few minutes, allow it to simmer before pouring it into the gravy dish. Rice, steamed vegetables, or roasted vegetables can be offered as a side dish.

Nutrition: Calories: 466.2, Proteins: 53.2 g, Carbs: 31 g, Fat: 13.4 g

7. Sweet Potato, Egg, and Avocado Breakfast

Preparation Time: 5 minutes

Cooking Time: 15 minutes

Servings: 1

Ingredients:

- Black pepper
- 2 tbsps. Coconut oil
- Salt
- ½ avocado
- 1 small sweet potato
- 2 medium chicken eggs

Directions:

This meal provides the optimal balance of nutrients to start you going that day and to keep you full for a longer time. Additionally, it is quite simple to prepare.

1. Peel and grate the sweet potato. You may also add shredded zucchini to your sweet potato dish.
2. Cook the sweet potatoes in a frying pan with medium-low heat. With salt and pepper, season the sweet potatoes and cook for 10 to 15 minutes or until the potato is soft. Regular stirring is required to keep the potatoes from scorching.
3. Remove the potato from the pan once it has reached the desired doneness. Break the eggs into the skillet one at a time after adding a little oil. Cook until the egg white has solidified.
4. Place the eggs and sweet potato on a plate and stir. Finally, peel and slice the avocado and serve.

Nutrition: Calories: 365, Proteins: 13 g, Carbs: 29 g, Fat: 15 g

8. Gingerbread Waffles

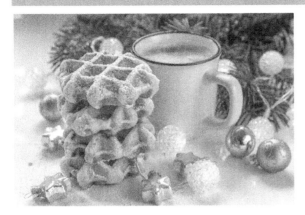

Preparation Time: 5 minutes

Cooking Time: 15 minutes

Servings: 6

Ingredients:

- ¼ c. pure maple syrup
- ½ c. almond or sunflower seed butter (unsweetened)
- ½ tsp. ground ginger
- 4 big eggs, room temperature
- 2 tbsps. Ghee or melted coconut oil
- ¼ tsp. sea salt
- 1 tbsp. molasses
- 3 tbsps. Coconut flour
- ¾ tsp. baking soda
- ⅓ c. almond milk or coconut milk
- 1 tsp. ground cinnamon
- 1 tbsp. Powdered arrowroot
- ½ tsp. ground cloves

Directions:

1. Preheat your waffle iron and put all of the ingredients in a blender.
2. Blend on low for 30 seconds, then high for 30 seconds, or until smooth.
3. To obtain a smooth mix, pause the blender and use a spatula to push the mixture down the sides.
4. If the waffle pan requires it, coat both sides with coconut oil. Carefully pour the batter into the waffle maker until it completely covers the bottom.
5. Cook for 45 seconds or until the waffle pan no longer steams. Each waffle pan may require a different amount of time to cook.

6. Rep till the entire mixture is finished. Serve warm with a piece of grass-fed butter and warmed maple syrup.

Nutrition: Calories: 327, Proteins: 5.2g, Carbs: 51.1g, Fat: 11.5g.

9. Bacon, Avocado, and Eggs

Preparation Time: 5 minutes

Cooking Time: 10 minutes

Servings: 1

Ingredients:

- ½ Avocado sliced
- 3 bacon rashers, choose organic
- 2 medium chicken eggs

Directions:

1. Heat the pan and add the bacon. Cook for 5-6 minutes or until the bacon is cooked to your liking.
2. Crack the eggs into a hot frying pan with a small amount of oil or half of the pan containing the bacon.
3. Cook until the egg yolk and whites are completely set.
4. Serve with avocado on the plate.

Nutrition: Calories: 680, Proteins: 41 g, Carbs: 16 g, Fat: 45 g

10. Smoked Salmon Frittata

Preparation Time: 10 minutes

Cooking Time: 10 minutes

Servings: 1

Ingredients:

- 2 chicken eggs
- 1 tsp. Dill chopped
- 1 tsp. Olive oil
- Sweet potatoes handful, roasted
- Black pepper to season
- Salt to season
- Courgettes (zucchini) handful, roasted
- Spinach handful, wilted
- 50g smoked salmon

Directions:

1. Prepare the grill for cooking over moderate heat.
2. Pour virgin olive oil into a big frying pan and heat it over medium heat. Cook the baked sweet potato, zucchini, and spinach in the pan.
3. Crack the eggs in a bowl and season with salt and pepper. Whisk them together with a fork until completely combined.
4. Break the reserved salmon into pieces and place them evenly on the vegetables. After that, place the eggs on top of the smoked salmon.
5. Allow the frittata to cook for about 5 minutes, or until it begins to firm, before placing the top of the dish under the grill for several minutes. Serve with chopped dill.

Note: If you want to create a big frittata to feed a larger number of people or have it for lunchtime over many days, you should use a larger frying pan and treble the amounts of each component.

Nutrition: Calories: 205, Proteins: 7.1 g, Carbs: 11.8 g, Fat: 10.6 g

11. Egg Bake

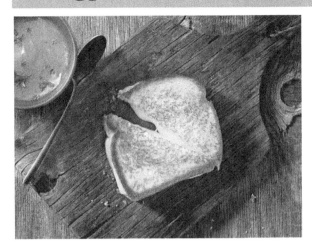

Preparation Time: 5 minutes

Cooking Time: 25 minutes

Servings: 2

Ingredients:

- 1 tbsp. pepper
- ¼ c. milk
- ½ c. cheddar
- 6 eggs
- 1 tbsp. salt
- 4 pieces of white bread

Directions:

1. Heat oven to 400°F. Use cooking spray on the pan to prevent it from sticking to the bottom and edges of the skillet.
2. Whisk the eggs until they are smooth. Stir in the pepper, milk, and salt.
3. To make a layer of bread alone, put torn pieces of white bread on the bottom of the pan.
4. Pour the eggs evenly over the bread. Push down to allow the bread to absorb all of the milk, eggs, and spices.
5. Spread a layer of cheese as a topping on the remaining ingredients.
6. Cook for 45 minutes at 400°F. Allow to cool down and enjoy.

Nutrition: Calories: 457, Proteins: 29 g, Carbs: 55.1 g, Fat: 12.9 g

12. Chocolate Zucchini Muffins

Preparation Time: 15 minutes

Cooking Time: 25 minutes

Servings: 12

Ingredients:

- ¾ tsp. ground cinnamon
- 4 big eggs
- ¾ c. zucchini, grated
- ½ c. non-dairy chocolate chips
- ½ c. maple syrup
- ¼ c. cacao powder
- ¼ tsp. sea salt
- 3 tbsps. arrowroot powder
- ½ tsp. ground nutmeg
- ⅓ c. coconut flour
- 1 ½ tsp. baking soda
- ½ c. apple sauce unsweetened
- 1 tbsp. Coconut oil for greasing

Directions:

1. Preheat the oven to 350°F. Prepare a muffin tray with baking cups or coconut oil.
2. Place the grated zucchini on a plate lined with paper towels to absorb moisture while making the batter.
3. Blend the eggs, applesauce, and maple syrup in a stand mixer on medium speed until fully combined.
4. Mix in the cacao powder, coconut flour, arrowroot powder, cinnamon, baking soda, sea salt, and nutmeg on medium speed again.
5. Wrap the zucchini in a paper towel and press it lightly to remove excess moisture. Fold in the zucchini and ¼ cup of the chocolate chips.
6. Fill each muffin cup two-thirds full of the prepared batter. Top with the remaining ¼ cup of chocolate chips. Cook for 22–25 minutes. Please wait 10 minutes before transferring it from the pan.

Nutrition: Calories: 111.6, Proteins: 1.2g, Carbs: 10.6g, Fat: 8.2g.

13. Egg, Turkey, and Cheese Breakfast Sandwich

Preparation Time: 2 minutes

Cooking Time: 2 minutes

Servings: 1

Ingredients:

- 1 sourdough bread
- 1 big egg
- ½ slice of mozzarella cheese
- 1 deli turkey breast slice (like Foster Farms)
- 1 tbsp. nonfat milk

Directions:

1. In a microwave-safe bowl, mix the egg and milk. Microwave for 30-45 seconds or until the mixture is firm but not dry.
2. Spread the cooked egg on one-half of the sourdough bread, followed by a folded turkey slice and cheese on top. Microwave the cheese for 30 seconds or until it achieves the appropriate consistency.
3. Place the remaining bread on top, and serve.

Nutrition: Calories: 268.1, Proteins: 19.1g, Carbs: 29.9g, Fat: 8.8g.

14. Breakfast Berry Crisp

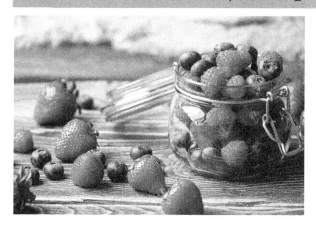

Preparation Time: 20 minutes

Cooking Time: 35 minutes

Servings: 10

Ingredients:

- ½ c. packed dark brown sugar
- ½ tsp. cinnamon
- 1 c. raw rolled oats
- 4 tsp. sugar
- ½ tsp. salt
- 1 c. blueberries
- 5 tbsps. butter mix
- 1 c. raspberries
- ⅓ c. almond flour
- ½ c. walnuts or pecans
- 2 c. halved fresh or frozen strawberries
- ¼ c. corn starch

Directions:

1. Set oven to 350°F.
2. Fill a large bowl with berries. Combine cornstarch and 4 tablespoons of Splenda or sugar in a mixing bowl. You will need to add more sugar if you use more sour berries. Place the mixture in a low-temperature oven.
3. In the same mixing bowl, combine the flour, oats, Splenda, brown sugar, almonds, salt, and cinnamon. Dice cold butter (for a vegan dish, replace it with a healthy oil such as walnut oil) and mix it into the ingredients until fully combined (it will seem to be a coarse meal).
4. Mix in the butter with your hands. Spread the topping evenly over the berries without pressing down.

31

5. Bake for 35 minutes, or until the berries burst and the top begins to brown, at 350°F. For dessert or brunch, serve with vanilla low-fat frozen yogurt or yogurt.

Nutrition: Calories: 198.1, Proteins: 40.7g, Carbs: 33.2g, Fat: 7.0g.

15. Muffins with Morning Glory

Preparation Time: 60 minutes

Cooking Time: 60 minutes

Servings: 12

Ingredients:

- ½ c. olive oil
- 1 tsp. ground cardamom
- ½ c. raisins
- ½ c. pure maple syrup
- 2 tsp. baking soda
- 3 big eggs
- ¼ c. unsweetened apple sauce
- 2 tsp. vanilla extract
- ½ c. crushed walnuts
- 1 c. carrots grated finely
- 1 tsp. ground ginger
- Cooking spray
- 2 c. almond flour
- 2 tsp. Ground cinnamon
- ¼ tsp. kosher salt

Directions:

1. Preheat the oven to 350°F. Line or grease 12 muffin tins with paper liners.
2. Mix baking soda, flour, cardamom, cinnamon, salt, and ginger in a large bowl and set aside.
3. In a separate bowl, combine applesauce, eggs, maple syrup, oil, and vanilla. Then, add the carrots.
4. Pour the liquid ingredients into the dry ingredients and stir until combined. Add the raisins and walnuts.
5. Distribute batter evenly into prepared muffin pans. Bake for 20 to 22 minutes, or until a toothpick inserted into the center of a muffin comes out mostly clean.
6. Allow 15 minutes to cool the muffin tray before removing and transferring it to a wire rack to cool completely. Place in an airtight container for 3-4 days or until frozen.

Nutrition: Calories: 264, Proteins: 5g, Carbs: 32g, Fat: 14g.

16. Golden Overnight Oats with Orange Flavor

Preparation Time: 6 hours 5 minutes

Cooking Time: 6 hours 5 minutes

Servings: 2

Ingredients:

- ¼ tsp. cinnamon, ground
- 2 tbsps. maple syrup, pure
- 1 c. rolled oats, old-fashioned
- Optional garnish: blueberries or raspberries, fresh
- ¼ tsp. kosher salt
- 1 tsp. Orange zest
- ¾ tsp. turmeric, ground
- 1 ¼ c. vanilla soymilk, unsweetened

Directions:

1. Mix all ingredients (excluding berries, if using) in a Mason jar or bowl; whisk thoroughly.
2. Refrigerate, covered, for 6 hours or overnight. Garnish with fresh berries if desired.

Nutrition: Calories: 263, Proteins: 9g, Carbs: 45g, Fat: 6g.

17. Blueberry Pancakes with Oatmeal

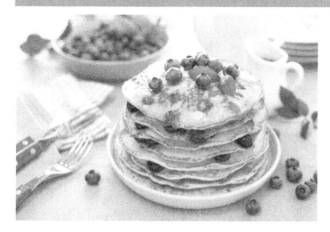

Preparation Time: 30 minutes

Cooking Time: 30 minutes

Servings: 3

Ingredients:

- ½ tsp. ground cinnamon
- 1 egg, whisked, big
- 1 tbsp. Olive oil
- ½ c. thawed frozen wild blueberries, plus more for garnish
- ¾ c. almond flour
- ¼ tsp. Salt
- ½ tsp. vanilla extract
- 2 tbsps. almond butter, creamy
- ¼ c. unsweetened cashew milk (or any non-dairy milk of your choice)
- 4 tbsps. Pure maple syrup, split
- Cooking spray
- 1 tsp. baking powder
- ½ c. oats for rapid cooking

Directions:

1. In a medium bowl, combine cashew milk and oats and let sit for 10 minutes.
2. Meanwhile, mix baking powder, flour, salt, and cinnamon, in a large bowl.
3. Stir egg, 1 tablespoon of oil, maple syrup, and vanilla into the oat mixture. Pour the oat mixture into the flour mixture, and whisk until incorporated. Next, fold in blueberries.
4. Preheat a greased nonstick skillet or pan over medium heat. While the skillet is heated, combine the remaining 3 tablespoons of almond butter and maple syrup on a small plate. Whisk in 1 tablespoon of boiling water until smooth. Place aside.

5. Pour a little less than ¼ cup of pancake batter onto a hot griddle per pancake. 2–3 minutes, or until the tops are studded with bubbles, and the edges appear dry and done. Cook for another 1 - 2 minutes on the other side. If desired, top with additional blueberries and almond butter sauce.

Nutrition: Calories: 392, Proteins: 10g, Carbs: 54g, Fat: 15g.

18. Green Peanut Butter-Banana Smoothie

Preparation Time: 5 minutes

Cooking Time: 5 minutes

Servings: 1

Ingredients:

- ¼ c. traditional rolled oats
- 1 medium thawed banana, cut
- 1 c. fresh spinach
- 1 c. vanilla soymilk, unsweetened
- 1 tbsp. salted peanut butter, natural
- ½ tsp. ground cinnamon

Directions:

1. Mix all ingredients in a high-powered blender until completely smooth.

Nutrition: Calories: 382, Proteins: 16g, Carbs: 51g, Fat: 14g.

19. Mediterranean Eggplant Shakshuka

Preparation Time: 25 minutes

Cooking Time: 25 minutes

Servings: 5

Ingredients:

- Crusty bread (optional)
- 3 minced cloves of garlic
- ¾ tsp. kosher salt, divided
- 5 big eggs
- 1 can of crushed tomatoes (15 oz.)
- 1 medium eggplant, cubed and sliced (no need to peel)
- 2 tbsps. virgin olive oil
- 3 tbsps. fresh chopped parsley
- 4 c. young spinach
- 2 tbsps. mild harissa paste
- ½ c. crumbled feta cheese, split (optional)

Directions:

1. Preheat the oven to 375 °F. Salt the eggplant with ¼ teaspoons and set it in a sieve. Let dry for 15 minutes.
2. In a large oven-safe skillet, heat the oil over medium heat. Cook for 7 to 8 minutes, occasionally stirring, until the eggplant is tender.
3. Cook for 2 minutes or until the spinach wilts and the garlic turns aromatic. Season with salt to taste.
4. Cook for 5 minutes, uncovered, with the tomatoes and harissa. Mix in half of the feta cheese if using.
5. In a skillet, gently crack eggs over tomatoes. Season the eggs with the remaining ¼ teaspoon salt, then sprinkle with the remaining feta cheese.
6. Place the frying pan in a preheated oven and bake for 10 minutes or until the eggs are barely set.
7. Garnish with parsley and serve with bread if desired.

Nutrition: Calories: 190, Proteins: 10g, Carbs: 15g, Fat: 11g.

20. Frittatas with Spinach and Red Peppers

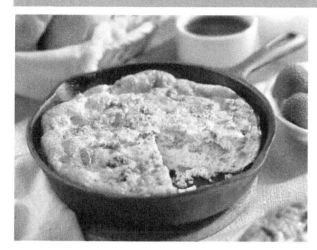

Preparation Time: 40 minutes

Cooking Time: 40 minutes

Servings: 6

Ingredients:

- 4 oz. fresh spinach
- 1 tsp. kosher salt
- ½ tsp. black pepper
- 12 big eggs
- 12 oz. chilled, unseasoned hash brown potatoes (or shredded, thawed chilled hash browns)
- Cooking spray
- 2 tsp. olive oil
- 1 red bell pepper sliced finely
- Freshly sliced avocados for serving (optional)

Directions:

1. Preheat oven to 400°F. Spread potatoes equally in 12 oiled muffin cups, pressing them into the bottoms and up the edges. Toast for 15 - 17 minutes or until golden brown.
2. Heat oil over medium heat in a large skillet, add bell pepper and simmer for 5 to 6 minutes or until softened.
3. Cook the spinach for 1 minute, stirring regularly until wilted. Spread the veggie mixture of equally overcooked potatoes in each muffin tin.
4. Combine the salt, eggs, and pepper in a large bowl, then spoon the mixture into each muffin cup. Put it in the oven again and cook it for 10 to 12 minutes or until the eggs are set.
5. Leave to cool for 5 minutes before removing from the pan. Serve with avocado slices, if preferred.

Nutrition: Calories: 219, Proteins: 15g, Carbs: 14g, Fat: 11g.

21: Avocado-Egg Salad Toast

Preparation Time: 10 minutes

Cooking Time: 10 minutes

Servings: 4

Ingredients:

- 1 tbsp. fresh lemon juice
- 1 big ripe avocado
- ½ tsp. kosher salt
- 4 sliced hard-boiled eggs
- ¼ tsp. black pepper
- 4 pieces of toasted white sourdough bread
- 1 tbsp. Minced fresh parsley + more for the season

Directions:

1. Remove the pit from the avocado and cut it in half. Remove the flesh from the skin and place it on a plate, mashing it thoroughly with a fork. Mix in the lemon juice, chopped eggs, salt, parsley, and pepper.
2. Distribute the mixture evenly over each piece of toasted bread. Garnish with additional parsley if desired.

Nutrition: Calories: 328, Proteins: 14g, Carbs: 38g, Fat: 14g

CHAPTER 4:
Lunch

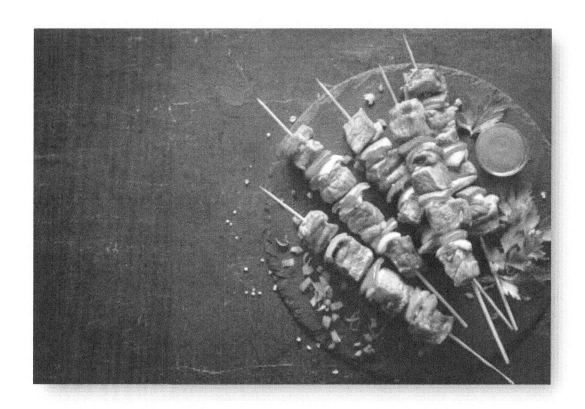

22. Chicken Lettuce Wraps

Preparation Time: 15 minutes

Cooking Time: 10 minutes

Servings: 5

Ingredients:

For the Chicken:

- 1¼ lb. ground chicken
- 1 tsp. fresh ginger, minced
- 2 tbsps. olive oil
- Salt and freshly ground black pepper to taste

For the Wraps:

- 10 romaine lettuce leaves
- 1½ c. carrot, peeled and julienned
- 2 tbsps. fresh parsley, chopped finely
- 2 tbsps. Fresh lime juice

Directions:

1. Heat the oil over medium heat in a skillet and sauté the ginger for about a minute.
2. Cook for 7-9 minutes, breaking the meat into smaller pieces with a wooden spoon, with the ground chicken, salt, and black pepper. Take the pan off the heat and set it aside to cool.
3. Place the lettuce leaves on individual serving dishes. Top each lettuce leaf with the cooked chicken, carrot, and cilantro. Serve immediately with a drizzle of lime juice.

Nutrition: Calories: 240; Fat: 15.1g; Carbs: 6.2g; Protein: 20.9g; Fiber: 2.34g

23. Beef Skewers

Preparation Time: 10 minutes

Cooking Time: 12 minutes

Servings: 5

Ingredients:

- 1½ lb. beef tenderloin, trimmed and cut into 1-inch cubes
- 2 tbsps. extra-virgin olive oil
- 2 tbsps. fresh lemon juice
- 1 tbsp. fresh thyme, chopped
- 1 tbsp. fresh oregano, chopped
- 1 tsp. lemon zest, grated
- Salt and ground black pepper to taste

Directions:

1. In a large mixing bowl, combine all ingredients except the meat cubes. Once all has been combined, add the meat cubes and generously coat them with the mixture.
2. Cover and place in the refrigerator to marinate overnight.
3. Preheat the grill to medium-high heat and coat with cooking spray.
4. Thread the beef cubes onto the pre-soaked bamboo skewers. Place the skewers on the grill for 10-12 minutes, flipping every 2-3 minutes. Serve right away.

Nutrition: Calories: 279; Fat: 5.2g; Carbs: 1g; Protein: 33g; Fiber: 0.2g

24. Roasted Pumpkin Curry

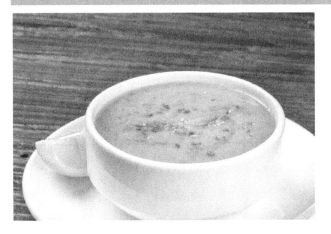

Preparation Time: 15 minutes

Cooking Time: 38 minutes

Servings: 4

Ingredients:

For Roasted Pumpkin:

- 1 medium sugar pumpkin, peeled and cubed
- 1 tsp. olive oil
- Salt to taste

For Curry:

- 2 large tomatoes, peeled, seeded, and chopped
- 2 c. homemade vegetable broth
- 2 tbsps. fresh parsley, chopped
- 1 tbsp. fresh lime juice
- 1 tsp. olive oil
- Salt and ground black pepper to taste

Directions:

1. Preheat the oven to 400°F and prepare a large baking sheet with parchment paper.
2. Toss together all of the roasted pumpkin fixings in a large mixing bowl. Place the pumpkin mixture in a single layer on the prepared baking sheet.
3. Cook for 20-25 minutes, flipping halfway through. Heat the oil in a large skillet over medium-high heat and sauté the tomatoes for about 2-3 minutes.
4. Allow the broth, salt, and black pepper to boiling. Reduce to low heat and cook for 10 minutes.
5. Cook for 10 minutes more after adding the roasted pumpkin and parsley. Serve immediately.

Nutrition: Calories: 76; Fat: 3.2g; Carbs: 9g; Protein: 2.1g; Fiber: 3.9g

25. Shrimp Maple Skewers

Preparation Time: 15 minutes

Cooking Time: 8 minutes

Servings: 4

Ingredients:

- 1 lb. medium raw shrimp, peeled and deveined
- ¼ c. olive oil
- 2 tbsps. fresh lime juice
- 1 tsp. Maple syrup
- ¼ tsp. ground cumin
- Salt and ground black pepper to taste

Directions:

1. In a large mixing bowl, combine all ingredients except the shrimp. Then, add the shrimp and thoroughly coat it with the herb mixture. Refrigerate for 30 minutes to marinate.
2. Preheat the grill to medium-high heat and oil the grill grate. Thread the shrimp onto pre-soaked wooden skewers.
3. Grill the skewers on a hot grill for 2-4 minutes per side. Remove from the oven and set aside for 5 minutes before serving.

Nutrition: Calories: 211; Fat: 15.2g; Carbs: 2.5g; Protein: 16g; Fiber: 0.7g

26. Pan-Seared Scallops

Preparation Time: 10 minutes

Cooking Time: 7 minutes

Servings: 4

Ingredients:

- 1¼ lb. fresh sea scallops, side muscles removed
- 2 tbsps. olive oil
- 1 tbsp. fresh parsley, minced
- Salt and ground black pepper to taste

Directions:

1. Sprinkle the scallops with salt and black pepper.
2. Heat the oil over medium-high heat in a large skillet and cook the scallops for about 2-3 minutes per side.
3. Stir in the parsley and serve hot.

Nutrition: Calories: 161; Fat: 7.8g; Carbs: 4.7g; Protein: 17.1g; Fiber: 0g

27. Shrimp Tomato Salad

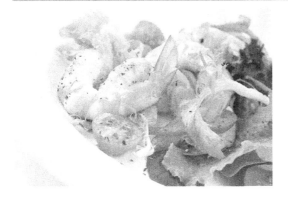

Preparation Time: 10 minutes

Cooking Time: 3 minutes

Servings: 5

Ingredients:

- 1 lb. shrimp, peeled and deveined
- 3 tomatoes, peeled, seeded, and sliced
- 1 lemon, quartered
- ¼ c. olives pitted
- ¼ c. fresh cilantro, chopped finely
- 2 tbsps. olive oil
- 2 tsp. fresh lemon juice
- Salt and ground black pepper to taste

Directions:

1. Bring a pan of lightly salted water to a boil with the quartered lemon. Cook the shrimp for 2-3 minutes or until pink and opaque.
2. Place the shrimp in a large bowl of icy water with a slotted spoon to stop the cooking process. Drain the shrimp thoroughly and pat dry with paper towels.
3. Add the oil, lemon juice, salt, and black pepper in a small mixing bowl.
4. Serve the shrimp, tomato, olives, and cilantro in individual dishes. Serve with the oil mixture drizzled on top.

Nutrition: Calories: 136; Fat: 7.6g; Carbs: 3.9g; Protein: 13.4g; Fiber: 1.7g

28. Tomato Salmon Bowl

Preparation Time: 10 minutes

Cooking Time: 0 minutes

Servings: 2

Ingredients:

- 6 oz. cooked salmon, chopped
- ¼ c. tomato, peeled, seeded, and chopped
- ¼ c. low-fat mozzarella cheese, cubed
- 1 tbsp. fresh dill, chopped
- 1 tsp. fresh lemon juice
- Salt, to taste

Directions:

1. In a medium bowl, add all the ingredients and stir to combine.
2. Serve immediately.

Nutrition: Calories: 186; Fat: 11.3g; Carbs: 1.1g; Protein: 20g; Fiber: 0.2g

29. Ground Chicken with Tomatoes

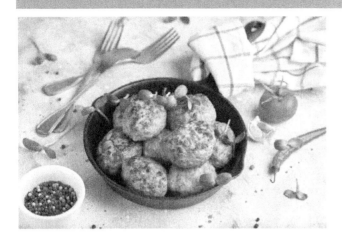

Preparation Time: 10 minutes

Cooking Time: 13 minutes

Servings: 4

Ingredients:

- 1¼ lb. ground chicken
- 2 tomatoes, peeled, seeded, and chopped
- 2 tbsps. olive oil
- 2 tbsps. fresh parsley, chopped
- Salt and ground black pepper to taste

Directions:

1. Heat oil over medium heat in a pan and cook the ground chicken for about 6-8 minutes.
2. Add the tomatoes and cook for about 4-5 minutes, stirring frequently. Stir in parsley, salt, and black pepper, and serve hot.

Nutrition: Calories: 274; Fat: 18.6g; Carbs: 2.6g; Protein: 25.3g; Fiber: 0.8g

30. Potatoes with Tomatoes

Preparation Time: 10 minutes

Cooking Time: 35 minutes

Servings: 6

Ingredients:

- 1½ lb. Yukon Gold potatoes, peeled and cubed
- 3 c. tomatoes, peeled, seeded, and chopped
- 1 c. water
- 2 tbsps. fresh lime juice
- 2 tbsps. olive oil
- Salt and ground black pepper to taste

Directions:

1. Heat oil over medium heat in a large skillet and cook the potatoes and tomatoes for about 4-5 minutes.
2. Add the water and simmer, covered within 20-30 minutes. Stir in the lime juice, salt, and black pepper and remove from the heat. Serve hot.

Nutrition: Calories: 89; Fat: 4.9g; Carbs: 11.2g; Protein: 1.7g; Fiber: 1.7g

31. Beef and Veggie Burgers

Preparation Time: 15 minutes

Cooking Time: 12 minutes

Servings: 8

Ingredients:

- 1 carrot, peeled and chopped finely
- 1 large beet, trimmed, peeled, and chopped finely
- 1 lb. lean ground beef
- 3 tbsps. olive oil
- 1 tbsp. fresh cilantro, chopped finely
- Salt and ground black pepper to taste

Directions:

1. Add all ingredients except oil to your large bowl and mix until well combined. Make equal-sized 8 patties from the mixture.
2. In a large non-stick sauté pan, heat the olive oil over medium heat and cook the patties in 2 batches for about 4-6 minutes per side. Serve hot.

Nutrition: Calories: 159; Fat: 8.8g; Carbs: 2g; Protein: 17.5g; Fiber: 0.4g

32. Liver with Onion and Parsley

Preparation Time: 15 minutes

Cooking Time: 22 minutes

Servings: 4

Ingredients:

- 1 lb. grass-fed beef liver, cut into ½-inch-thick slices
- ½ c. fresh parsley
- 3 tbsps. olive oil, divided
- 2 large onions, sliced
- 2 tbsps. freshly squeezed lemon juice
- Salt and ground black pepper to taste

Directions:

1. Heat 1 tablespoon of oil in a large skillet over high heat. Sauté the onions and salt for around 5 minutes. Reduce the heat to medium, cook for another 10-15 minutes, and then set aside.
2. Heat an additional tablespoon of oil in the same skillet. Heat the oil over medium-high heat. Season the liver with salt and black pepper. Cook for about 1-2 minutes or until browned.
3. Cook for another 1-2 minutes or until browned.
4. Heat the remaining oil in the skillet over medium heat. Stir in the sautéed onion, parsley, and lemon juice. Cook for approximately 2-3 minutes.
5. Serve the onion mixture over the liver right away.

Nutrition: Calories: 274; Fat: 14g; Carbs: 11.8g; Protein: 24g; Fiber: 1.4 g

33. Egg and Avocado Endive Wraps

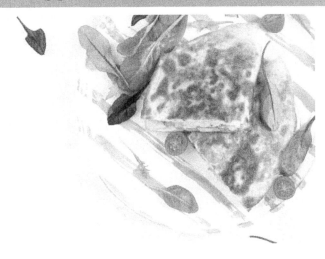

Preparation Time: 20 minutes

Cooking Time: 0 minutes

Servings: 5

Ingredients:

- 4 organic hard-boiled eggs, peeled and finely chopped
- 4-5 endive bulbs
- 2 cooked turkey bacon slices, chopped
- 1 ripe avocado, peeled, pitted, and chopped
- 1 tbsp. freshly squeezed lemon juice
- 1 tbsp. fresh parsley, chopped
- 2 tbsps. celery stalk, chopped
- Salt and freshly ground black pepper to taste

Directions:

1. In a bowl, mash the avocado and lemon juice until smooth. Add the celery, parsley, eggs, salt, and black pepper and mix well.
2. Split the endive leaves and divide the avocado mixture over the endive leaves evenly. Top with bacon and serve immediately.

Nutrition: Calories: 183; Fat: 11.1g; Carbs: 12.7g; Protein: 10.9g; Fiber: 1g

34. Greek Cucumber Salad

Preparation Time: 10 minutes

Cooking Time: 0 minutes

Servings: 4

Ingredients:

- 4 medium cucumbers, peeled, seeded, and chopped
- ½ c. nonfat Greek yogurt
- 1½ tbsp. fresh dill, chopped
- 1 tbsp. fresh lemon juice
- Salt and freshly ground black pepper to taste

Directions:

1. In a large bowl, mix all the ingredients until well combined.
2. Serve immediately.

Nutrition: Calories: 54; Fat: 0.8g; Carbs: 8.6g; Protein: 4.5g; Fiber: 1g

35. Beef and Spinach Burgers

Preparation Time: 15 minutes

Cooking Time: 12 minutes

Servings: 4

Ingredients:

- 1 egg, beaten
- 1 lb. lean ground beef
- 1 c. fresh baby spinach leaves, chopped
- ½ c. sun-dried tomatoes, peeled, seeded, and chopped
- ¼ c. low-fat feta cheese, crumbled
- 2 tbsps. olive oil
- Salt and ground black pepper to taste

Directions:

1. Add all the ingredients except oil to a large bowl and mix until well combined. Make 4 equal-sized patties from the mixture.
2. In a cast-iron pan, heat oil over medium-high heat and cook the patties for about 5-6 minutes per side until the desired doneness. Serve immediately.

Nutrition: Calories: 259; Fat: 17.1g; Carbs: 1.5g; Protein: 25.6g; Fiber: 0.7g

36. European Beet Soup

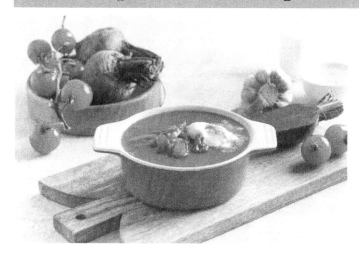

Preparation Time: 10 minutes

Cooking Time: 5 minutes

Servings: 3

Ingredients:

- 2 c. beets, trimmed, peeled, and chopped
- 2 c. fat-free yogurt
- 4 tsp. fresh lemon juice
- 2 tbsps. fresh dill
- 1 tbsp. fresh chives, minced
- Salt to taste

Directions:

1. In a high-speed blender, blend all the ingredients except the chives until smooth.
2. Transfer the soup to a pan over medium heat and cook for about 3-5 minutes until heated.
3. Serve immediately with a garnish of chives.

Nutrition: Calories: 122; Fat: 0.2g; Carbs: 14.6g; Protein: 16g; Fiber: 2.6g

37. Pasta with Asparagus

Preparation Time: 10 minutes

Cooking Time: 10 minutes

Servings: 4

Ingredients:

- 1 lb. asparagus, trimmed and cut into 1½-inch pieces
- ½ lb. cooked hot pasta, drained
- 2 tbsps. olive oil
- Salt and freshly ground black pepper to taste

Directions:

1. In a large cast-iron skillet, heat the oil over medium heat and cook the asparagus, salt, and black pepper for about 8-10 minutes, stirring occasionally.
2. Place the hot pasta and toss to coat well. Serve immediately.

Nutrition: Calories: 171; Fat: 7.7g; Carbs: 21.1g; Protein: 5.3g; Fiber: 2.9g

38. Versatile Mac 'n Cheese

Preparation Time: 15 minutes

Cooking Time: 8-9 minutes

Servings: 3

Ingredients:

- 2 c. refined elbow macaroni, cooked and drained
- 1½ lb. butternut squash, peeled, cubed
- 1 c. low-fat Swiss cheese, shredded
- ⅓ c. low-fat milk
- 1 tbsp. olive oil
- Salt and freshly ground black pepper to taste

Directions:

1. In a pan of boiling water, cook the squash cubes for about 6 minutes or until tender. Return the squash cubes to the same pan after draining.
2. Mash the squash with a fork and set aside on low heat. Cook for about 2-3 minutes, constantly stirring, after adding the cheese and milk.
3. Mix in the macaroni, oil, salt, and black pepper. Remove from the heat and serve immediately.

Nutrition: Calories: 322; Fat: 7.7g; Carbs: 44.6g; Protein: 17.3g; Fiber: 1.9g

39. Turkey Burgers

Preparation Time: 15 minutes

Cooking Time: 16 minutes

Servings: 5

Ingredients:

- 1 lb. lean ground turkey
- 5 oz. low-fat Halloumi cheese, grated
- 2 eggs
- 1 tbsp. fresh rosemary, chopped finely
- 1 tbsp. fresh parsley, chopped finely
- Salt and ground black pepper to taste

Directions:

1. Preheat the grill to medium-high heat and oil the grill grate.
2. Mix all of the ingredients in a large mixing basin until well blended. Form the ingredients into 10 equal-sized patties.
3. Place the burgers on the grill and cook for 5-8 minutes per side or until fully cooked.

Nutrition: Calories: 208; Fat: 10.3g; Carbs: 1g; Protein: 28g; Fiber: 0.2g

40. Pasta With Zucchini and Tomatoes

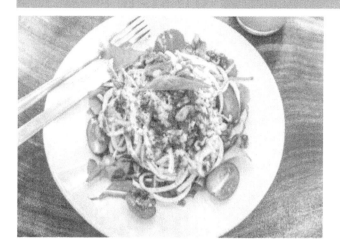

Preparation Time: 15 minutes

Cooking Time: 20 minutes

Servings: 8

Ingredients:

- 3 tomatoes
- 1 lb. refined pasta
- 1 lb. zucchini, peeled, seeded, and sliced
- ¾ c. low-fat feta cheese, crumbled
- ¼ c. olive oil
- 1 tbsp. garlic
- 1 tsp. dried oregano, crushed
- Salt to taste
- Water, as needed

Directions:

1. Add tomatoes to a large pan of salted boiling water and cook for about 1 minute. Transfer the tomatoes to a bowl of ice water with a slotted spoon.
2. Add the pasta to the same pan of boiling water and cook for about 8-10 minutes. Drain the pasta well.
3. Meanwhile, peel the blanched tomatoes, remove the seeds, and chop them finely.
4. Heat the oil over medium heat in your large skillet and sauté the zucchini and garlic for about 4-5 minutes.
5. Add the tomatoes and oregano and cook for about 3-4 minutes. Add the pasta and cheese and stir to combine. Serve hot.

Nutrition: Calories: 272; Fat: 10.5g; Carbs: 25.3g; Protein: 9.5g; Fiber: 1.3g

41. Beef and Mozzarella Burgers

Preparation Time: 15 minutes

Cooking Time: 10 minutes

Servings: 2

Ingredients:

- 8 oz. lean ground beef
- 1 oz. part-skim mozzarella cheese, cubed
- 1 tbsp. olive oil
- Salt and ground black pepper to taste

Directions:

1. In a mixing bowl, combine the meat, salt, and black pepper until well incorporated. Form the ingredients into 2 equal-sized patties.
2. Insert a mozzarella cube into each burger and top with the beef.
3. Heat the oil in a frying pan over medium heat and cook the patties for about 3-5 minutes per side. Serve immediately.

Nutrition: Calories: 311; Fat: 16.6g; Carbs: 0.5g; Protein: 38.4g; Fiber: 0g

42. Tuna Stuffed Avocado

Preparation Time: 10 minutes

Cooking Time: 0 minutes

Servings: 2

Ingredients:

- 1 large avocado, halved and pitted
- 1 (5- oz.) can of water-packed tuna, drained and flaked
- 3 tbsps. fat-free plain yogurt
- 2 tbsps. fresh lemon juice
- 1 tsp. fresh parsley, chopped finely
- Salt and ground black pepper to taste

Directions:

1. Cut an avocado in half and remove around 2-3 tablespoons of flesh from each avocado. Arrange the avocado halves on a dish and drizzle each with 1 teaspoon of lemon juice.
2. Transfer the avocado flesh to a bowl and set aside. Stir in the tuna, yogurt, parsley, lemon juice, salt, and black pepper.
3. Divide the tuna mixture evenly between the 2 avocado halves. Serve right away.

Nutrition: Calories: 215; Fat: 11.8g; Carbs: 7g; Protein: 20.6g; Fiber: 3.2g

43. Shrimp Lettuce Wraps

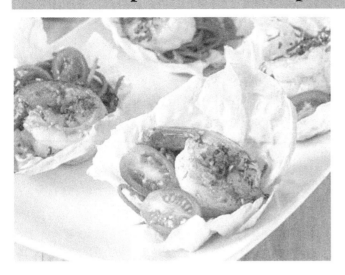

Preparation Time: 10 minutes

Cooking Time: 4 minutes

Servings: 6

Ingredients:

- 1½ lb. shrimp, peeled, deveined, and chopped
- 12 butter lettuce leaves
- 1 c. carrot, peeled and julienned
- 1 tbsp. extra-virgin olive oil
- Salt and ground black pepper to taste

Directions:

1. In a large pan, heat the oil over medium heat and cook the shrimp with salt and black pepper for about 3-4 minutes. Set aside.
2. Arrange the lettuce leaves onto serving plates. Place the shrimp over the leaves evenly and top with carrot. Serve immediately.

Nutrition: Calories: 164; Fat: 4.3g; Carbs: 3.8g; Protein: 26g; Fiber:0.5g

44. Fried Rice with Kale

Preparation Time: 10 minutes

Cooking Time: 12 minutes

Servings: 2

Ingredients:

- 3 sliced scallions
- 1 ½ c. cooked white rice
- 1 c. kale, stemmed and chopped
- 2 tbsps. stir-fry sauce
- 1 tbsp. Extra-virgin olive oil

Directions:

1. In a large skillet over medium-high heat, heat the olive oil. Stir in the scallions and greens. Cook the vegetables until they are soft.
2. In a mixing bowl, combine the stir-fry sauce and brown rice. Cook, often stirring, until completely heated. Serve!

Nutrition: Calories: 308; Fat: 11.3g; Carbs: 41.9g; Protein: 9.5g; Fiber: 4.38 g

45. Shrimp and Tomato Bake

Preparation Time: 15 minutes

Cooking Time: 27 minutes

Servings: 6

Ingredients:

- 1½ lb. large shrimp, peeled and deveined
- ½ c. homemade chicken broth
- 2 c. tomatoes, peeled, seeded, and chopped
- ¼ c. fresh parsley, chopped
- 4 oz. low-fat feta cheese, crumbled
- 2 tbsps. olive oil
- ¾ tsp. Dried oregano, crushed

Directions:

1. Preheat oven to 350°F. Heat the oil in a sauté pan over medium-high heat and sauté the shrimp and oregano for about 2 minutes.
2. Stir in the parsley and salt and distribute evenly into a casserole dish.
3. In the same pan, boil the broth over medium heat for about 2-3 minutes or until reduced by half. Cook for about 2-3 minutes after adding the tomatoes.
4. Spread the tomato mixture equally over the shrimp mixture and top with cheese.
5. Bake for 15-20 minutes or until the top is golden brown. Serve immediately.

Nutrition: Calories: 150; Fat: 7g; Carbs: 5.4g; Protein: 25.7g; Fiber: 0.9g

46. Lemony Scallops

Preparation Time: 10 minutes

Cooking Time: 5 minutes

Servings: 4

Ingredients:

- 1 lb. sea scallops
- 2 tbsps. olive oil
- 2 tbsps. fresh rosemary, chopped
- 1 tbsp. Fresh lemon juice
- ½ tsp. lemon zest, grated
- Salt and ground black pepper to taste

Directions:

1. In a medium sauté pan, heat the oil over medium-high heat and sauté the rosemary and lemon zest for about 1 minute.
2. Add the scallops and cook within 2 minutes per side. Stir in lemon juice, salt, and black pepper, and serve hot.

Nutrition: Calories: 166; Fat: 8.1g; Carbs: 3.9g; Protein: 19.2g; Fiber: 0.7g

CHAPTER 5:
Dinner

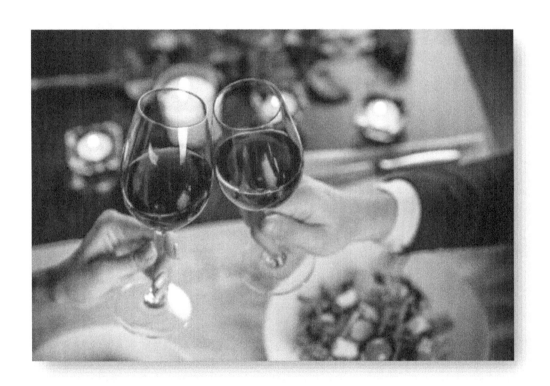

47. Stuffed Zucchini Boats

Preparation Time: 15 minutes

Cooking Time: 30 minutes

Servings: 3-6

Ingredients:

- 1 lb. ground turkey
- 1 (28 oz.) can crush tomatoes
- 6 large zucchinis, divide half lengthwise and scoop out the seeds
- 2 garlic cloves minced
- 1 small yellow onion, diced
- 4 oz. Mozzarella cheese, shredded
- 1 oz. Parmesan cheese, freshly grated
- ½ tbsp. olive oil
- ¼ tsp. garlic powder
- Flat-leaf parsley for garnishing
- Kosher salt and ground black pepper to taste
- Cooking spray

Directions:

1. Preheat the oven to 425°F and spray a 9x13-inch baking dish with cooking spray.
2. Season the zucchini with salt, pepper, and garlic powder after brushing it with olive oil. Roast for 20 minutes in the preheated dish or until it softens.
3. In the meantime, sauté the onions and garlic in a large skillet over medium-high heat.
4. Cook for 3-4 minutes before adding the ground turkey and browning it. Allow the tomatoes to come to a boil.
5. Reduce the heat to medium and cook until the zucchini is tender. Season with salt and pepper to taste.
6. Bake for 5 minutes or until the mozzarella cheese melts. Garnish with Parmesan cheese and parsley, and serve hot.

Nutrition: Calories: 173; Fat: 17.1g; Carbs: 10.5g; Protein: 14.2g; Fiber: 3.6g

48. Chicken Cutlets

Preparation Time: 10 minutes

Cooking Time: 5 minutes

Servings: 4

Ingredients:

- 1 lb. chicken breast cutlets
- ¼ c. refined white flour
- 4 tsp. red wine vinegar
- 2 tsp. minced garlic cloves
- 2 tsp. dried sage leaves
- 2 tsp. olive oil
- Salt and pepper to taste

Directions:

1. Place a plastic wrap on the kitchen surface and sprinkle with half of the sage, garlic, and vinegar mixture.
2. Spread the remaining vinegar mixture over the chicken breast and wrap it in plastic. Season with pepper and salt to taste.
3. Use the second piece of plastic wrap to wrap the chicken. Pound the breast with a kitchen mallet until it is flattened. Allow it to stand for 5 minutes.
4. Coat your chicken in flour on both sides.
5. Heat the oil in a skillet over medium heat. Cook for 12 minutes or until half of the chicken breast is browned on the bottom.
6. Cook for 3 minutes on the other side. Remove the cutlets, set them aside, and repeat with the remaining cutlets.

Nutrition: Calories: 189; Fat: 5.5g; Carbs: 6.63g; Protein: 26.4g; Fiber: 0.2g

49. Halibut Curry

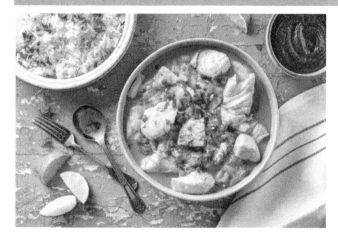

Preparation Time: 10 minutes

Cooking Time: 9 minutes

Servings: 2

Ingredients:

- 1 lb. halibut, skin and bones removed, cut into 1-inch pieces
- ½ (14 oz.) canned coconut milk
- 2 c. no-salt-added chicken broth
- 1 tbsp. extra-virgin olive oil
- 1 tsp. Ground turmeric
- ⅛ tsp. ground black pepper
- 1 tsp. Curry powder
- ¼ tsp. sea salt

Directions:

1. Heat the olive oil in a non-stick skillet over medium-high heat.
2. Mix the curry powder and turmeric in a bowl. To bloom the spices, cook for 2 minutes in your skillet, stirring continuously.
3. Stir in the halibut, coconut milk, chicken broth, pepper, and salt. Adjust to medium-low heat and let it simmer. Cook for 6-7 minutes until the fish is opaque. Serve!

Nutrition: Calories: 373; Fat: 31g; Carbs: 5g; Protein: 21.6g; Fiber: 1g

50. Rosemary Chicken

Preparation Time: 15 minutes

Cooking Time: 20 minutes

Servings: 2

Ingredients:

- 1 lb. chicken breast tenders
- 1 tbsp. chopped fresh rosemary leaves
- 1 tbsp. Extra-virgin olive oil
- ⅛ tsp. Ground black pepper
- ¼ tsp. sea salt

Directions:

1. Preheat the oven to 425°F.
2. Set the chicken tenders on a baking sheet with a rim. Brush them with oil, and sprinkle them with salt, rosemary, and pepper oil.
3. Bake for 15-20 minutes until the juices run clear. Serve!

Nutrition: Calories: 336; Fat: 13.1g; Carbs: 0.3g; Protein: 51g; Fiber: 0.1g

51. Lemony Salmon

Preparation Time: 10 minutes

Cooking Time: 14 minutes

Servings: 4

Ingredients:

- 4 (6-oz.) boneless, skinless salmon fillets
- 1 tbsp. fresh lemon zest, grated
- 2 tbsps. extra-virgin olive oil
- 2 tbsps. fresh lemon juice
- Salt and freshly ground black pepper to taste

Directions:

1. Preheat your grill to medium-high heat and lightly oil the grill grate.
2. Mix all of the ingredients except the salmon fillets in a medium bowl. Add the salmon fillets and generously cover them with the garlic mixture.
3. Cook the salmon fillets on the grill for about 6-7 minutes per side. Serve immediately.

Nutrition: Calories: 383; Fat: 27g; Carbs: 0.9g; Protein: 34.5g; Fiber: 0.2g

52. Herbed Salmon

Preparation Time: 10 minutes + marinating time

Cooking Time: 8 minutes

Servings: 4

Ingredients:

- 4 (4-oz.) salmon fillets
- ¼ c. olive oil
- 2 tbsps. fresh lemon juice
- 1 tsp. dried oregano, crushed
- 1 tsp. dried basil, crushed
- Salt and freshly ground black pepper to taste

Directions:

1. In a large mixing bowl, combine all ingredients except the salmon. Add the salmon and generously coat it with the marinade.
2. Cover and place in the fridge for at least 1 hour to marinate. Preheat the grill to medium-high heat and coat the grill grate with cooking spray.
3. Cook the fish for about 4 minutes per side on the grill. Serve immediately.

Nutrition: Calories: 341; Fat: 27.6g; Carbohydrates: 1.0g; Protein: 23g; Fiber: 0.3g

53. Cantaloupe Gnocchi

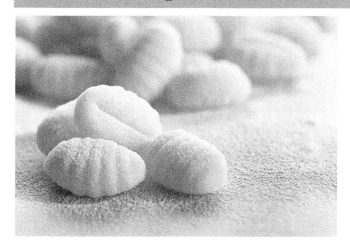

Preparation Time: 10 minutes

Cooking Time: 4-6 minutes

Servings: 4

Ingredients:

- 4-5 c. cantaloupe, skinned, cut into chunks, and steamed
- 2 c. refined flour
- 1 tsp. olive oil
- Himalayan salt to taste
- Water, as needed

Directions:

1. Combine the cooked cantaloupe and flour in a large mixing basin. Stir and knead thoroughly to make a doughy mixture. Set aside several gnocchi-shaped pieces made with your hands.
2. Boil some water, add your gnocchi and simmer for 4-6 minutes or until they float on top. Drain well and serve!

Nutrition: Calories: 305; Fat: 2.2g; Carbs: 58.1g; Protein: 9.1g; Fiber: 2.2g

54. Veggie Risotto

Preparation Time: 10 minutes

Cooking Time: 23 minutes

Servings: 2

Ingredients:

- 1 c. white risotto rice, cooked
- 1 c. grated zucchini, peeled and deseeded
- 1 c. water
- ½ c. canned green beans halved
- 1 tbsp. extra virgin olive oil
- 1 tsp. apple cider vinegar
- 1 tsp. dried basil
- A sprig of parsley, finely chopped
- Himalayan salt to taste
- Herbs for garnish

Directions:

1. Within 6-8 minutes, fry the vegetables in the oil in your skillet until they begin to color and soften.
2. Combine the apple cider vinegar, herbs, rice, and water in a mixing bowl. Cook for 15 minutes or until the flavor is to your liking. Garnish with herbs before serving.

Nutrition: Calories: 142; Fat: 3.4g; Carbs: 25.5g; Protein: 2.9g; Fiber: 1.3g

55. Lemon Pepper Turkey

Preparation Time: 10 minutes

Cooking Time: 20 minutes

Servings: 4

Ingredients:

- 1 lb. turkey breasts, boneless and skinless halved
- 2 lemons, divided (1 zested and 1 sliced)
- 2 minced cloves of garlic
- ½ c. refined flour
- ½ c. chicken broth
- 4 tbsps. olive oil
- 1 tbsp. lemon pepper seasoning
- 1 tsp. kosher salt

Directions:

1. Preheat the oven to 400°F.
2. Mix 1 lemon zest, flour, salt, and pepper in a bowl. Coat the turkey thoroughly.
3. On 1 side, bake the turkey for 5 minutes in heated oil.
4. Bake for 15 minutes, or until done, with the remaining ingredients. Serve.

Nutrition: Calories 231; Fat 6g; Carbs 12g; Protein 14g; Fiber 1.7g

56. Chicken Piccata

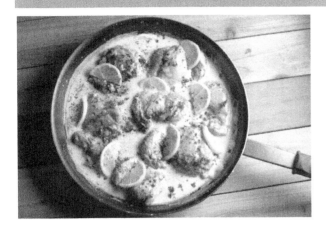

Preparation Time: 10 minutes

Cooking Time: 20 minutes

Servings: 4

Ingredients:

- 3 chicken breasts sliced into 6 cutlets
- 2 garlic cloves minced
- 2 lemons' juice
- 1 lemon, sliced
- 2 c. chicken stock
- 1 c. almond flour
- ¼ c. capers
- ⅓ c. white wine
- 6 tbsps. olive oil
- Granulated garlic, to taste
- Salt and pepper to taste

Directions:

1. Season the cutlets with salt, pepper, and granulated garlic. Cover them in flour.
2. Heat the olive oil in a skillet and fry the chicken cutlets for 4 minutes per side. Serve it on a platter.
3. Brown the garlic in the same skillet, then add the lemon slices, granulated garlic, salt, pepper, stock, lemon juice, and wine.
4. Allow it to boil, add the capers and chicken, and cook for 5 minutes. Serve.

Nutrition: Calories 276; Fat 15g; Carbs 14g; Protein 17g; Fiber 1g

57. Whole Roasted Trout

Preparation Time: 10 minutes

Cooking Time: 16 minutes

Servings: 2

Ingredients:

- ½ lb. whole trout
- 1 lemon, sliced
- 6 sprigs of fresh thyme
- ½ shallot, thinly sliced
- 1 tbsp. olive oil
- 4 tsp. butter, cubed (if tolerated)
- Salt and black pepper to taste

Directions:

1. Preheat the oven to 425°F.
2. Season the fish with salt and pepper after coating it with oil.
3. Place on an aluminum-lined baking sheet, skin side down, and top with the other ingredients.
4. Bake for 12-16 minutes before serving.

Nutrition: Calories 178; Fat 6g; Carbs 13g; Protein 14.3g; Fiber 2g

58. Turkey and Kale Sauté

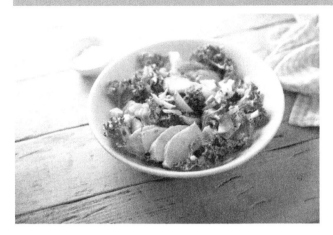

Preparation Time: 15 minutes

Cooking Time: 35 minutes

Servings: 2

Ingredients:

- 1 lb. ground turkey breast
- 3 minced garlic cloves
- ½ chopped onion
- 1 c. stemmed and chopped kale
- ½ tsp. sea salt
- 1 tbsp. extra-virgin olive oil
- 1 tbsp. fresh thyme leaves
- A pinch of freshly ground black pepper

Directions:

1. In a large nonstick skillet, heat the olive oil over medium-high heat.
2. Combine the turkey, onion, kale, thyme, pepper, and salt in a mixing bowl. Cook the turkey for 5 minutes, crumbling it with a spoon until it is browned.
3. Cook for 30 minutes, constantly stirring, after adding the garlic. Serve!

Nutrition: Calories: 342; Fat: 9.58g; Carbs: 7g; Protein: 58.7g; Fiber: 1.6g

59. Winter Apple Poke Bowl

Preparation Time: 10 minutes

Cooking Time: 50 minutes

Servings: 2

Ingredients:

- 1 packet of precooked white rice
- 1 red apple, peeled and sliced
- ½ butternut pumpkin, peeled, seeded, and chopped
- 7 oz. diced halloumi
- ½ c. parsley and coriander
- ½ c. chopped chives
- 2 tbsps. lemon juice
- 2 tbsps. olive oil
- 1 tbsp. organic honey
- 1 tsp. grated ginger

Directions:

1. Preheat the oven to 390°F. Cook for 30-40 minutes or until the pumpkin is soft. Cook the halloumi till brown in a pan.
2. Combine the remaining ingredients in a bowl, then top with halloumi and roasted pumpkin. Serve!

Nutrition: Calories 178; Fat 4g; Carbs 14g; Protein 3g; Fiber 4g

60. Prawn and Tomato Spaghetti

Preparation Time: 20 minutes

Cooking Time: 6 minutes

Servings: 6

Ingredients:

- 20 green prawns, peeled and deveined
- 6 tomatoes, peeled, seeded, and chopped
- 4 garlic cloves, sliced
- 13 oz. refined spaghetti, cooked and drained
- 2 tbsps. chopped parsley leaves
- 1 tbsp. olive oil

Directions:

1. Sauté the garlic in your pan with hot oil for 1 minute over medium heat.
2. Add the prawns and cook within 2 to 3 minutes. Add tomatoes and cook for 2 minutes.
3. Toss in the parsley and pasta until well combined. Serve!

Nutrition: Calories 490; Fat 6.5g; Carbs 50g; Protein 33g; Fiber 1.2g

61. Chicken Cacciatore

Preparation Time: 10 minutes

Cooking Time: 20 minutes

Servings: 2

Ingredients:

- 1 lb. skinless chicken, cut into bite-size pieces
- 1 (28 oz.) can of crushed tomatoes, drained
- ¼ c. black olives, chopped
- 1 tbsp. Extra-virgin olive oil
- ½ tsp. Onion powder
- ½ tsp. Garlic powder
- ¼ tsp. sea salt
- A pinch of freshly ground black pepper

Directions:

1. In a nonstick skillet, heat the olive oil over medium-high heat. Cook until the chicken is golden brown.
2. Stir in the tomatoes, garlic powder, olives, salt, onion powder, and pepper. Cook for 10 minutes, stirring occasionally. Serve!

Nutrition: Calories: 343; Fat: 14.2g; Carbs: 20.2g; Protein: 39g; Fiber: 5.1g

62. Peach Stew

Preparation Time: 10 minutes

Cooking Time: 10 minutes

Servings: 6

Ingredients:

- 5 c. peeled and cubed peaches
- 2 c. water
- 3 tbsps. stevia
- 1 tsp. grated ginger

Directions:

1. Combine the peaches, stevia, ginger, and water in a pot.
2. Toss well, cook for 10 minutes over medium heat, divide into bowls and serve cold.

Nutrition: Calories 142; Fat 1.5g; Carbs 7.8g; Protein 2.4g, Fiber 1.7g

63. Shrimp Salmon Tomato Stew

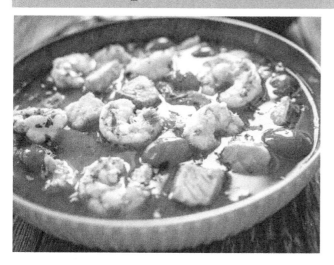

Preparation Time: 10 minutes

Cooking Time: 18 minutes

Servings: 8

Ingredients:

- 1 lb. salmon fillets, cubed
- 1 lb. shrimp, peeled and deveined
- 4 c. fish bone broth
- 2½ c. fresh tomatoes, peeled, seeded, and chopped
- 2 tbsps. fresh lime juice
- 3 tbsps. fresh parsley, chopped
- Salt and freshly ground black pepper to taste

Directions:

1. In a large soup pot, combine the tomatoes and broth and boil. Reduce the heat to medium and continue to cook for about 5 minutes.
2. Simmer for 3-4 minutes after adding the salmon. Cook for about 4-5 minutes after adding the shrimp.
3. Remove from heat and stir in the lemon juice, salt, and black pepper. Serve immediately with a garnish of parsley.

Nutrition: Calories: 173; Fat: 5.5g; Carbs: 3.2g; Protein: 27.1g; Fiber: 0.7g

64. Zero-Fiber Chicken Dish

Preparation Time: 5 minutes + marinating time

Cooking Time: 10 minutes

Servings: 6

Ingredients:

- 4 (6-oz.) chicken breast halves, boneless, skinless
- 2 tbsps. olive oil
- Salt and freshly ground black pepper to taste

Directions:

1. Season each chicken breast with salt and black pepper.
2. Place the chicken breast halves on a rimmed baking sheet over a rack. Refrigerate for at least 30 minutes before serving. Remove from the oven and blot dry with paper towels.
3. Heat the oil in a skillet over medium-low heat. Cook the chicken breast halves, smooth-side down, for 9-10 minutes without moving them.
4. Cook for another 6 minutes or until the chicken breasts are fully cooked. Allow cooling before slicing and serving!

Nutrition: Calories: 178; Fat: 7.7g; Carbs: 0.1g; Protein: 26g; Fiber: 0g

65. Easiest Tuna Salad

Preparation Time: 15 minutes

Cooking Time: 0 minutes

Servings: 4

Ingredients:

For the Dressing:

- 2 tbsps. fresh dill, minced
- 2 tbsps. olive oil
- 1 tbsp. fresh lime juice
- Salt and freshly ground black pepper to taste

For the Salad:

- 2 (6-oz.) cans of water-packed tuna, drained and flaked
- 6 hard-boiled eggs, peeled and sliced
- 1 c. tomato, peeled, seeded, and chopped
- 1 large cucumber, peeled, seeded, and sliced

Directions:

1. Add all the ingredients for the dressing to a bowl and whisk until well blended.
2. In another large serving bowl, add all the ingredients for the salad and mix well.
3. Divide the tuna mixture onto serving plates. Drizzle with dressing and serve.

Nutrition: Calories: 277; Fat: 14.5g; Carbs: 5.9g; Protein: 31.2g; Fiber: 0.96g

66. Brazilian Fish Stew

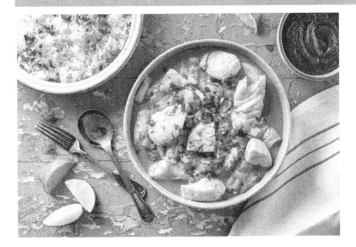

Preparation Time: 10 minutes

Cooking Time: 19 minutes

Servings: 4

Ingredients:

- 1 to 1 ½ lb. firm white fish
- 1 lime's juice and zest
- ½ tsp. salt

For the Sauce:

- 4 garlic cloves, chopped
- 1 onion, diced
- 1 red bell pepper, chopped (if tolerated)
- 1 (14 oz.) can of coconut milk
- 1 ½ c. chopped tomatoes, no seeds and peeled
- 1 c. carrot, diced
- 1 c. chicken stock
- ½ c. chopped herbs
- 2 to 3 tbsps. olive oil
- 1 tbsp. tomato paste
- ½ tsp. salt
- 1 tsp. ground cumin

Directions:

1. Coat the fish in lime juice, zest, and salt.

2. Sauté the onion and salt in a pan for 2 to 3 minutes. Cook for 4 to 5 minutes with the carrot, garlic, and bell pepper.
3. After adding the stock, spices, and tomato paste, cook for 5 minutes. Cook for 4 to 6 minutes after adding the coconut milk and the fish. Serve!

Nutrition: Calories 404; Fat 19.7g; Carbs 12.6g; Protein 44g; Fiber 1.2g

67. Turkey with Rosemary

Preparation Time: 15 minutes

Cooking Time: 10 minutes

Servings: 2

Ingredients:

- 1 lb. boneless, skinless turkey breasts cut into bite-size pieces
- 2 minced garlic cloves
- ½ chopped onion
- 2 tbsps. extra-virgin olive oil
- 1 tbsp. chopped fresh rosemary leaves
- ¼ tsp. sea salt
- A pinch of freshly ground black pepper

Directions:

1. Heat the olive oil over medium-high heat in a nonstick skillet or pan.
2. Combine the onion, rosemary, turkey, salt, and pepper in a mixing bowl. Cook until the turkey is done and the vegetables are tender. Cook for 30 seconds more after adding the turkey.

Nutrition: Calories: 413; Fat: 17g; Carbs: 6.8g; Protein: 54g; Fiber: 1.6g

68. Grilled Salmon Steaks

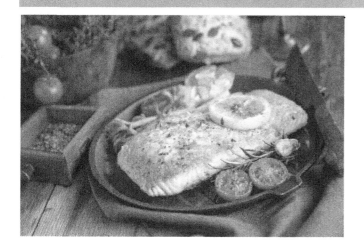

Preparation Time: 5 minutes

Cooking Time: 10 minutes

Servings: 2

Ingredients:

- 1 tsp. olive oil
- 2 salmon steaks
- 2 tbsps. soy sauce

Directions:

1. Preheat the grill and grease the grates.
2. Brush the sauce over the fish fillets and cook for 5 minutes per side. Serve!

Nutrition: Calories 295; Fat 17g; Carbs 7g; Protein 31g; Fiber 0g

69. Fiesta Chicken Tacos

Preparation Time: 10 minutes

Cooking Time: 6 minutes

Servings: 8

Ingredients:

- 1 lb. chicken breast, skinless and boneless, cut into thin strips
- 8 well-tolerated corn tortillas, heated
- 1 c. each sliced red bell pepper and red onion (if tolerated)
- 1 c. mixed salad greens
- 1 tbsp. olive oil
- ½ tsp. ground cumin
- ¼ tsp. salt

Directions:

1. Season the chicken with cumin and sauté for 3 minutes in a pan with heated oil.
2. For 3 minutes, sauté the onion and bell pepper in 1 teaspoon of oil. Put the chicken back in the pan and season with salt.
3. Fill each tortilla with the chicken mixture and 2 tablespoons of mixed greens. Secure with a roll and serve.

Nutrition: Calories 320; Fat 6.4g; Carbs 36.1g; Protein 30.3g; Fiber 3.8g

70. Shrimp Scampi Pizza

Preparation Time: 10 minutes

Cooking Time: 20 minutes

Servings: 8

Ingredients:

- 1 (13.8 oz.) pack of refined pizza dough
- 1 lb. peeled shrimp, cooked and sliced
- 2 c. shredded mozzarella
- 1 tbsp. cornmeal
- ½ c. ricotta cheese
- 6 cloves of roasted garlic
- 1 tbsp. dried basil
- Cooking spray

Directions:

1. Preheat the oven to 400°F and coat a baking pan with cooking spray.
2. Place the dough in the baking pan and stretch it over the cornmeal. Cook for 8 minutes.
3. In a mixing dish, combine the ricotta and garlic. Spread this on top of the dough. Combine the shrimp, mozzarella, and basil in a mixing bowl.
4. Bake for 12 minutes, then remove from the oven and serve!

Nutrition: Calories 175; Fat 5g; Carbs 18.7g; Protein 14g; Fiber 1g

71. Duck with Pear

Preparation Time: 10 minutes

Cooking Time: 60 minutes

Servings: 2-3

Ingredients:

- 2 organic duck breasts
- 1 c. canned pear
- ¼ c. coconut oil
- 2 tbsps. garlic minced (if tolerated)
- ¼ c. honey
- 1 sprig of rosemary (if tolerated)
- 2 portions of lettuce leaves
- Himalayan salt to taste

Directions:

1. In a skillet, heat the coconut oil and whisk in the rosemary, garlic, honey, and Himalayan salt. Cook for around 2 minutes.
2. Meanwhile, preheat the oven to 375°F and line a baking sheet with parchment paper.
3. Coat the duck breasts in the mixture and place them on a baking sheet. Cook for 60 to 75 minutes or until well done. Serve!

Nutrition: Calories: 540; Fat: 23g; Carbs: 36g; Protein: 24g; Fiber: 1.2g

CHAPTER 6:
Dessert

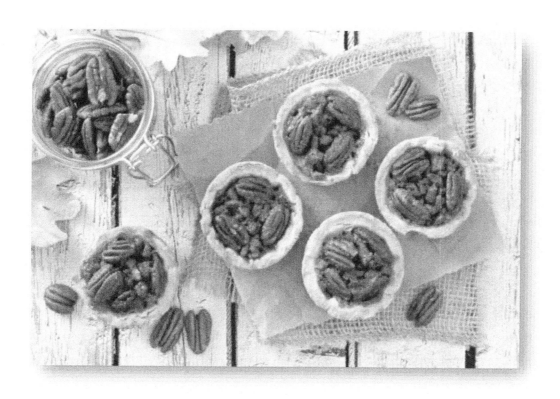

72. Vegan Pecan Tart with Chocolate Crust

Preparation Time: 15 minutes

Cooking Time: 0 minutes

Servings: 10

Ingredients:

- 1 c. dates
- ¼ c. cacao powder
- 1 tbsp. coconut oil
- 1 c. pecans
- ¼ c. maple syrup
- 1 ½ c. raw cashews
- 1 tsp. vanilla
- 2 tbsps. coconut oil
- ¼ c. cacao powder
- Pecans to garnish
- A pinch of Salt
- 2 - 3 tbsps. water
- ½ c. chocolate chips

Directions:

1. Put the cashews in a bowl and cover them in at least one-inch of boiling water for 1 hour.
2. Make the crust while the cashews soak by filling a food processor halfway with nuts, cacao powder, dates, and coconut oil and processing on high speed until a firm dough forms. Flatten the mixture into a tart pan.
3. Drain and rinse the cashews. Mix 2 tablespoons of water with melted white chocolate, unsweetened chocolate, coconut oil, syrup, vanilla, and salt. Blend low until creamy and smooth (it should be thick but pourable).
4. Fill the crust with the filling and top with additional pecans if desired. Freeze for at least 2 hours, preferably overnight.
5. Let rest for 10 minutes before serving. After, cut it up and enjoy!

Nutrition: Calories: 309, Protein: 6 g, Carbs: 27 g, Fat: 23 g

73. Vegan Granola Cups

Preparation Time: 5 minutes

Cooking Time: 25 minutes

Servings: 12

Ingredients:

- 3 tbsps. coconut oil
- Yogurt
- Sliced strawberries
- 6 tbsps. almond butter
- ¾ c. maple syrup
- Chia seeds
- Pinch of sea salt
- Sliced kiwi/mango
- 3 tbsps. flaxseed meal
- 1 tsp. cinnamon
- Fresh blueberries/blackberries
- 3 c. rolled oats
- Sprinkle of coconut

Directions:

1. Preheat the oven to 350°F. Set aside a 12-cup muffin tray greased with nonstick spray.
2. Combine all the ingredients for the granola cup. The "batter" should be firm.
3. Fill each muffin cup with ¼ cup of an oat mixture.
4. Press the oat mix into the middle and up the right side of each cup using damp fingertips to cover as many cups as possible while leaving a well in the center.
5. Fill every cup with yogurt and fruit of your choosing! If preferred, top with jojoba seeds and coconut.

Nutrition: Calories: 222, Protein: 5 g, Carbs: 30 g, Fat: 4 g

74. Dairy- and Gluten-Free Carrot Cake

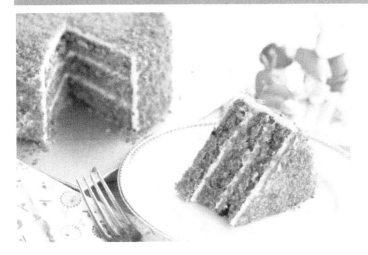

Preparation Time: 10 minutes

Cooking Time: 40 minutes

Servings: 4

Ingredients:

- 200g cream cheese
- 250g carrots grated
- 2 tsp. Bicarbonate of soda
- 60g walnuts (optional)
- 160g almond flour
- 2 chicken eggs
- 25g spread
- 1 tsp. Cinnamon ground
- 180ml olive oil
- 180g sugar, caster

Directions:

1. Preheat the oven to 160°C. In a mixing bowl, thoroughly incorporate all of the cake ingredients except the carrots and walnuts.
2. Combine the carrots with the rest of the ingredients.
3. Bake the batter for 1 hour and 5 minutes, or until a knife inserted into the center of the cake comes out clean.
4. Next, using a mixer, combine dairy-free spread, dairy-free cream cheese, and sugar to make the frosting. When you don't want the frosting to be overly sweet, reduce the amount of sugar.
5. Apply the frosting to the cake after it has cooled. This ganache is runny in the dairy-free version!

Nutrition: Calories: 390, Proteins: 7.8 g, Carbs: 14.4 g, Fat: 35.7 g

75. Free Dairy Banana Chocolate Ice Cream

Preparation Time: 60 minutes

Cooking Time: 0 minutes

Servings: 2

Ingredients:

- 2 bananas
- ½ tbsp. Honey
- 1 tbsp. Cocoa powder

Directions:

1. In a blender, combine the banana chunks. Blend until the bananas are almost foamy.
2. Mix in the chocolate powder and honey. Freeze for several hours in an airtight (sealed) container/jar.
3. Serve on its own or with berries. If you prefer sweeter ice cream, add a little more honey.

Nutrition: Calories: 111, Proteins: 1.6 g, Carbs: 27.9 g, Fat: 0.5 g

76. Gluten- and Dairy-Free Blueberry Cupcakes with Lemon Icing

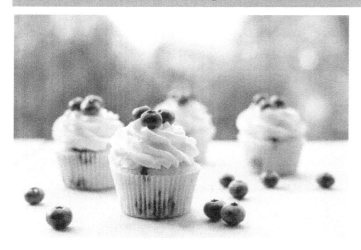

Preparation Time: 15 minutes

Cooking Time: 15 minutes

Servings: 3

Ingredients:

- 110g sugar
- 2 tsp. Coconut milk
- 2 chicken eggs
- 110g free dairy spread
- 450g icing sugar
- Blueberries approx. 2 handfuls
- 110g almond flour
- 4 tbsps. Lemon juice
- 1 tsp. Vanilla extract

Directions:

1. Preheat a microwave to 180°C (350°F).
2. Combine the dairy-free spread and sugar for several minutes using a hand mixer or a blender.
3. In a mixing bowl, combine the eggs with a metal fork. For a few seconds, combine a spoonful of egg and a tablespoon of flour with the butter and sugar combination.
4. Add another spoonful of egg and flour until the egg is completely incorporated. This helps to keep the mixture from curdling. Add any remaining flour and thoroughly mix it up.
5. Mix in the fresh coconut milk and vanilla extract briefly.
6. Add the blueberries and mix them in by hand.

7. After dividing the batter evenly among 12 cupcake liners, place it in the saucepan for 10 to 15 minutes. They should be golden in color and bouncy to the touch when finished.

8. When adding frosting, add the lemon juice to a bowl and sift in the powdered sugar while mixing. Continue to add icing sugar until the mixture is thick and dribble-resistant.

9. After the cakes have cooled, ice them and top them with a blueberry. Refrigerate the cakes for the icing to set.

Nutrition: Calories: 271, Proteins: 4 g, Carbs: 24 g, Fat: 18 g

77. Free Dairy Chocolate Hazelnut Spread

Preparation Time: 5 minutes

Cooking Time: 0 minutes

Servings: 4

Ingredients:

- 1 tbsp. Maple syrup
- 3 tbsps. Coconut milk
- 2 tbsps. Cocoa powder
- Hazelnuts almonds

Directions:

1. Place hazelnuts in a food processor or mixer and pulse until finely ground.
2. Blend the remaining ingredients until the mixture is smooth. You will need to add more coconut milk to the mixture to thin it down.
3. To make it more chocolaty, add more cocoa powder; to make it gentler/sweeter, use more maple syrup.
4. Serve with pancakes, toast, fresh fruit, or whatever else you choose.

Nutrition: Calories: 79, Proteins: 8.4 g, Carbs: 35 g, Fat: 4.4 g

78. Tofu Chocolate Cake

Preparation Time: 15 minutes

Cooking Time: 30 minutes

Servings: 16

Ingredients:

- 1-300g block of dessert/soft tofu
- 1 package ultra-moist chocolate cake mix
- ¼ c. water

Directions:

1. Combine cake mix and tofu in a blender or food processor (I use a hand/stick blender).
2. When everything is blended, add a quarter cup of water and blend until smooth.
3. Place in a baking dish and bake according to the directions on the cake mix packaging, considering the type of dish used. I sometimes make cupcakes and other times a square cake.

Note: DO NOT ADD THE EGG, OIL, OR ANY OTHER INGREDIENTS REQUIRED BY THE CAKE MIX; the tofu will replace them.

Nutrition: Calories: 189.5, Proteins: 2.9g, Carbs: 35.8g, Fat: 4.0g.

79. Pink Lemonade Pie

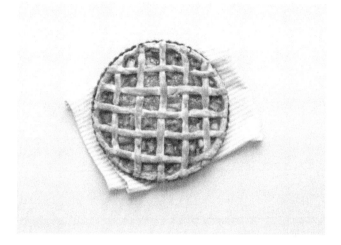

Preparation Time: 5 minutes

Cooking Time: 240 minutes

Servings: 16

Ingredients:

- 2 small containers of Cool Whip Lite
- 2 Premade Graham Cracker Pie Crusts
- ½ can Minute Maid Frozen Pink Lemonade Concentrated
- 1 can Eagle Brand Fat-Free Sweetened Condensed Milk

Directions:

This frozen dessert requires no cooking time, simply time in the freezer; it is often prepared in the morning so that it may freeze before dinner's dessert course.

1. Mix the pink lemonade, milk, and one container of cool whip.
2. Fill the 2 crusts with the ingredients.
3. Top with the remaining Cool Whip. Freeze for at least 3 hours, covered.

Nutrition: Calories: 281.6, Proteins: 3.0g, Carbs: 46.9g, Fat: 9.7g.

80. Autumnal Vegan Carrots with Walnuts

Preparation Time: 5 minutes

Cooking Time: 10 minutes

Servings: 2

Ingredients:

- 1 tsp. cinnamon
- ½ tsp. nutmeg
- ⅛ c. raisins
- ¼ c. sugarless syrup
- 1 ½ c. sliced carrots

Directions:

1. Boil the carrots until they are tender.
2. Combine the remaining ingredients.
3. Stir over low heat until the syrup thickens and the carrots are coated. Serve and have fun!!

Nutrition: Calories: 168.4, Proteins: 3.5g, Carbs: 19.4g, Fat: 10.1g.

81. Java Bananas

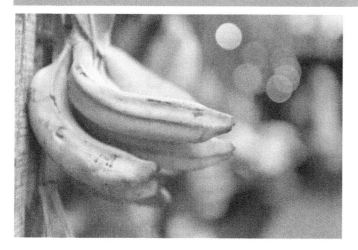

Preparation Time: 5 minutes

Cooking Time: 25 minutes

Servings: 2

Ingredients:

- 6 tbsps. dark brown sugar
- 1 tbsp. butter
- 2 tsp. vanilla extract
- 3 bananas, peeled and sliced into half-inch pieces
- 6 tbsps. brewed espresso

Directions:

1. Melt the butter with the vanilla in a big saucepan.
2. After the brown sugar has been combined, add the banana slices.
3. Cook, occasionally stirring, over medium-high heat until the bananas begin to crackle.
4. Cook until the liquids condense into a thick syrup after adding the coffee.
5. Don't mix the bananas. Tilt the skillet and pour the sauce over the bananas as they cook.
6. Serve as a treat on its own or as a topping for vanilla yogurt or ice cream.

Nutrition: Calories: 394.7, Proteins: 2.2g, Carbs: 88.1g, Fat: 6.7g.

82. Sweet Dessert Bliss

Cooking Time: 10 minutes

Servings: 4

Ingredients:

- Fruit, if preferred
- 4 tbsps. Nonfat whipped topping
- Fat-free or low-fat plain yogurt
- 1 packet of Splenda, if desired
- 1 package of sugarless gelatin

Directions:

1. Prepare and chill 1 packet of gelatin.
2. When the gelatin is cool, combine it with 1 low-fat or fat-free yogurt container and whipped topping. Refrigerate for another hour after fully mixing.
3. Serve and have fun!

Nutrition: Calories: 56.9, Proteins: 4.6g, Carbs: 6.4g, Fat: 1.0g.

83. Free Gluten and Dairy Apple Crumb

Preparation Time: 10 minutes

Cooking Time: 25 minutes

Servings: 4

Ingredients:

- 175g almond flour
- 135g sugar
- 110g spread
- 3 medium apples Bramley

Directions:

1. Preheat the oven to 190°C.
2. Toss the apples with 2 tablespoons of sugar and arrange them in an oven-safe dish. You want a lot of layers of apples.
3. In a mixing dish, combine the remaining sugar, flour, and dairy-free spread (or butter) to make a crumbly mixture.
4. Pour the mixture over the apples and gently press.
5. Place in the oven for 45 minutes or until the top has solidified and begins to brown.
6. Serve with non-dairy custard or ice cream if desired.

Nutrition: Calories: 213, Proteins: 2 g, Carbs: 31.8 g, Fat: 9.6 g

84. Custard Dairy Free

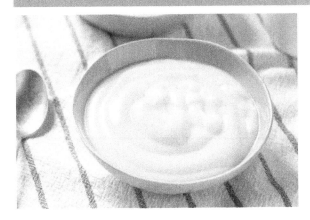

Preparation Time: 10 minutes

Cooking Time: 0 minutes

Servings: 4

Ingredients:

- 2 chicken yolk eggs only
- 15g caster sugar
- 300ml almond milk
- ¼tsp. Vanilla extract
- 1 tsp. almond flour

Directions:

1. Mix the sugar, egg yolk, and cornstarch in a mixing bowl.
2. Bring the milk and vanilla extract to a simmer in a saucepan over medium heat.
3. Return the mixture to heat after adding the milk to the egg mixture. Stir until the sauce thickens.
4. If you want a thicker custard, mix 1 tablespoon of cold water with an additional teaspoon of cornstarch and stir it into the custard. While the custard is heating, the cornstarch will thicken it.
5. Serve immediately! This custard goes great with apple crumble, which is gluten-free and dairy-free.

Nutrition: Calories: 44, Proteins: 1.2 g, Carbs: 10.3 g, Fat: 0.1 g

85. Fried Honey Bananas

Preparation Time: 4 minutes

Cooking Time: 4 minutes

Servings: 2

Ingredients:

- 1 tbsp. Coconut oil
- 1 tsp. Cinnamon (optional)
- 1 tbsp. Honey
- 1 banana sliced

Directions:

1. Mix the honey and 1-2 tablespoons of warm water in a mixing bowl.
2. Place the pan on the burner after adding the oil and heating it over medium heat.
3. Once the pan is hot, add the bananas and cook on each side for 1 to 2 minutes.
4. Remove the pan from the heat and pour the honey and water mixture over the apples, followed by the cinnamon.
5. Allow cooling slightly before serving.

Nutrition: Calories: 370, Proteins: 2 g, Carbs: 52 g, Fat: 20 g

86. Avocado Sorbet

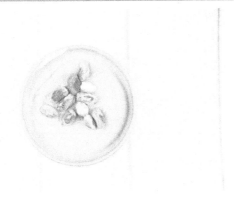

Preparation Time: 15 minutes

Cooking Time: 15 minutes

Servings: 4

Ingredients:

- ½ c. Agave syrup
- ½ c. Mild coconut milk
- 2 tbsps. Organic lime peel
- ⅔ to ¾ c. Avocado, chopped into chunks (1 medium avocado)
- ¼ c. Fresh lemon juice (from 2 to 3 limes)

Directions:

1. Blend the avocado in a mixer until it is almost entirely smooth. Add the agave syrup, scrape down the sides, and purée.
2. While the machine is running, slowly pour the coconut milk and combine until smooth. Blend in the lemon juice and zest until completely blended and smooth.
3. Place the mixture in a storage container and chill for at least 4 hours and up to 1 day or until well chilled.
4. Using an ice cream machine, make the avocado sorbet mixture according to the manufacturer's directions. If you like a soft texture, serve immediately; if you prefer a firmer texture, chill for at least 6 hours or up to 1 day.

Nutrition: Calories: 150, Proteins: 1g, Carbs: 25g, Fat: 5g.

87. Banana Cupcakes

Preparation Time: 20 minutes

Cooking Time: 40 minutes

Servings: 4

Ingredients:

- Almond flour
- 1 c. Warm water
- ½ c. Almond meal
- Ripe bananas
- 2 free-range eggs
- 2 tbsps. Honey

Directions:

1. Preheat the ovens to 375°F.
2. Grease a muffin tray with butter or olive oil and set aside.
3. Whisk everything together in a large mixing bowl.
4. After whisking the eggs, slowly drizzle in the honey and water. Finally, add the cut bananas.
5. Cook for about 25 minutes or until a toothpick can be inserted and retrieved with no residue attached.
6. Allow for 10 minutes of cooling on a rack.

Nutrition: Calories: 120, Proteins: 34 g, Carbs: 5 g, Fat: 1 g

88. Flourless Cake

Preparation Time: 30 minutes

Cooking Time: 40 minutes

Servings: 4

Ingredients:

- 1 c. Ground hazelnuts
- 1 tbsp. Sugar
- Butter to grease the pan
- Powdered sugar
- 200 g of bitter chocolate
- 4 eggs
- 1 heaping spoon of cocoa powder
- 150 g of butter

Directions:

1. In a bain-marie, melt the chocolate and butter. Remove the pan from the heat and set it aside to cool.
2. Whisk the eggs and sugar together. Mix in the cocoa powder then whisks once more.
3. While whisking, include the ground hazelnuts. Butter a springform pan with a diameter of 21 cm.
4. Place parchment on the bottom of the pan, then grease the top and bottom of the parchment. Bake for thirty minutes at 190°C in a preheated oven.
5. Remove from the oven and set aside for 10 minutes before serving.
6. With a spatula or a knife, loosen both sides of the cake, then place it on a serving plate. Sprinkle powdered sugar on top, then serve.

Nutrition: Calories: 250, Proteins: 15 g, Carbs: 34 g, Fat: 2 g

89. Eggless Honey Cake

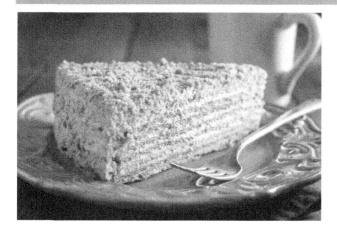

Preparation Time: 40 minutes

Cooking Time: 30 minutes

Servings: 6

Ingredients:

- 125 ml honey
- 250 ml milk
- ½ tsp. Baking soda
- ½ tsp. Baking powder
- 125g butter
- 4 chopped figs
- 230g of almond flour
- 100g cane sugar
- 20g of cocoa powder
- ½ tsp. Cinnamon powder

Directions:

1. Grease a baking sheet and preheat the oven to 185 °C.
2. Melt the butter and set it aside.
3. Sieve all of the dry ingredients, such as cinnamon powder, baking powder, baking soda, and flour are all included. Honey, milk, and cane sugar should also be combined.
4. Add the melted butter and diced figs into the mixture with a whisk.
5. After pouring the batter onto the baking sheet, bake for 10 to 15 minutes.
6. Cool completely before serving.

Nutrition: Calories: 160, Proteins: 32 g, Carbs: 28 g, Fat: 2 g

90. Christmas in a Cup

Preparation Time: 40 minutes

Cooking Time: 30 minutes

Servings: 6

Ingredients:

- Free-range eggs
- 1 tsp. Ground cinnamon
- ½ tsp. Ground cloves
- 1 tsp. Baking powder
- 1 tbsp. Stevia or your preferred sweetener
- ½ tsp. Ground ginger
- 125g of almond flour
- 75g butter

Directions:

1. Whisk the eggs and combine them with the remaining ingredients in a mixing bowl.
2. After that, stir in the melted butter.
3. Place the batter in paper muffin liners and bake for 10 to 15 minutes at 180°C.
4. Insert a skewer, or something similarly long and thin, into the center of the cake and remove it to see if the cupcakes are baking.
5. When the cake sticks to the skewer, the ingredients have not yet been set, and the cakes require additional baking time.

Nutrition: Calories: 200, Proteins: 25 g, Carbs: 15 g, Fat: 3 g

91. Brownie Bites

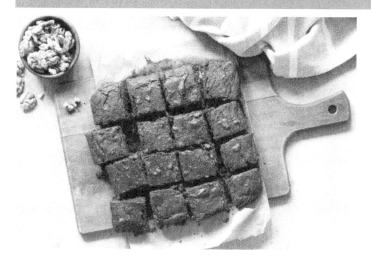

Preparation Time: 20 minutes

Cooking Time: 30 minutes

Servings: 4

Ingredients:

- ¼ Tsp. Kosher salt
- ¼ c. Almond butter
- 1 tbsp. Cocoa powder
- ½ c. Hazelnuts
- ½ c. Raw cashews
- Pitted Medjool dates
- ½ tsp. Vanilla extract

Directions:

1. In a food processor, finely chop the dates, cashews, and hazelnuts.
2. Process until the almond butter, chocolate powder, vanilla extract, and salt form a clump.
3. Chill 1 tablespoon of the mixture balls and let rest until ready to eat.
4. Refrigerate in an airtight container for up to 2 weeks after opening.

Nutrition: Calories: 180, Proteins: 30 g, Carbs: 85 g, Fat: 10 g

92. Blueberry Galette

Preparation Time: 30 minutes + 4 hours chilling time

Cooking Time: 45 minutes

Servings: 8

Ingredients:

For the Pastry:

- ¼ c. + 3 tbsps. Arrowroot powder
- 5 tbsps. Cold unsalted grass-fed butter
- 2 ¼ c. Cashew flour
- 1 tbsp. Coconut flour
- ¼ c. Pure maple syrup
- ¼ tsp. Sea salt

For the Filling:

- 1 lemon zest
- 2 c. Blueberries
- 1 tbsp. Coconut sugar
- 1 tbsp. Maple syrup
- 1 ½ tsp. Fresh lemon juice
- 2 tsp. Arrowroot powder

For the Egg Wash:

- 1 tbsp. Full-fat coconut milk

- 1 big egg yolk

Directions:

1. In a food processor, combine the arrowroot, cashew flour, sea salt, and coconut flour for 15 seconds.
2. Mix in the maple syrup for 15 seconds or until the mixture is crumbly and well combined.
3. Add 1 tablespoon of cold butter at a time, pulsing the food processor between additions, until the butter is pea-sized and the dough begins to come together.
4. Form the ingredients into a tight ball and flatten it with your palms into a disc. Wrap it tightly in plastic wrap and place it in the refrigerator to cool for 4 hours.
5. After the dough has cooled, preheat the oven to 325°F.

6. Place the dough between 2 pieces of parchment paper on a level surface. Form the dough into a 12-inch-diameter circle with a thickness of about 12 inches. Transfer the parchment paper and dough to a baking sheet.

7. Gently combine the filling ingredients in a mixing bowl.

8. Place the filling in the center of the folded-out dough. Fold the crust's edges so that about 2 inches of dough extends beyond the perimeter of the filling. Fill up any holes or fissures that exist.

9. Whisk together the egg yolk and coconut milk. Spread the egg wash over the crust's surface with a pastry brush. Bake the galette for 45 minutes or until the crust is golden brown. Serve!

Nutrition: Calories: 282, Proteins: 0.6g, Carbs: 17g, Fat: 24.2g.

93. Royal Crown Pie

Preparation Time: 60 minutes

Cooking Time: 60 minutes

Servings: 8

Ingredients:

- ½ 8-ounce container of Cool Whip Free, thawed
- 1 four-serving packet of Jell-O Sugar-Free Strawberry Gelatin dessert mix
- 1 four-serving packet of Jell-O Sugar-Free Strawberry Banana Gelatin dessert mix
- ½ 8-ounce container of frozen Cool Whip Free
- 1 four-serving packet of Jell-O Sugar-Free Lime Gelatin dessert mix
- 1 four-serving packet of Jell-O Sugar-Free Orange Gelatin dessert mix

Directions:

1. In a medium mixing bowl, combine the orange mix and 1 cup of boiling water for at least 2 minutes (until completely dissolved). Then, put the mixture in a medium-sized rectangle or square container. Place the container in the fridge. Continue with the remaining Jell-o and refrigerate until set (about 4 hours or overnight).
2. Slide a knife down the edges of each container to remove the gelatins once they have solidified. Refrigerate each item after cutting it into half-inch cubes.'
3. In a large mixing bowl, whisk together the strawberry mix and 1 cup of boiling water for at least 2 minutes (until completely dissolved). Then, add half a cup of cold water and place the bowl in the refrigerator. Allow 45 minutes to chill (till slightly thickened but still thoroughly blendable).
4. In the meantime, line a 9-inch pie pan or rectangle dish with 10 crackers. (For a tight fit, you may need to trim them halfway.)
5. When the Strawberry Jell-O has thickened, rapidly whisk in the Cool Whip (if you have one). Slowly fold the chunks into the Cool Whip/Jell-O mixture.
6. Using nonstick cooking spray, lightly mist the edges of the cake pan, holding the crust. Pour everything into a pan and refrigerate until firm.

Nutrition: Calories: 67.3, Proteins: 2.7g, Carbs: 7.8g, Fat: 1.5g.

94. Mocha Ricotta Crème

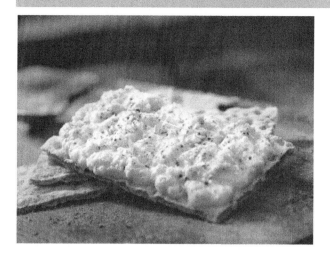

Preparation Time: 10 minutes

Cooking Time: 10 minutes

Servings: 1

Ingredients:

- ¼ tsp. Vanilla extract
- ½ c. Part-skimmed ricotta
- Splash espresso powder (or instant coffee)
- ½ tsp. Unsweetened cocoa powder
- 5 tiny chocolate chips
- 1 packet of sugar-replacement

Directions:

1. Combine the ricotta, chocolate powder, vanilla essence, and sugar replacement in a dessert dish.
2. Serve cooled with an espresso powder coating and chocolate chunks on top.

Nutrition: Calories: 200.5, Proteins: 14.5g, Carbs: 10.7g, Fat: 11.2g.

95. Orange Muffins

Preparation Time: 30 minutes

Cooking Time: 30 minutes

Servings: 6

Ingredients:

- ½ c. Orange juice
- ½ tsp. Grated orange rind
- ⅓ c. Protein powder
- ½ tsp. Baking soda
- ¼ tsp. Salt
- 1 tbsp. Butter or coconut oil
- 1 tbsp. Honey
- ⅔ c. almond flour
- 1 egg

Directions:

1. In a large mixing bowl, combine the flour mixture, protein isolate, baking soda, salt, sugar, and orange rind.
2. Use a fork or a whisk to combine them.
3. Pour the oranges, crack the egg, and measure out the oil. The mixture should be stirred. It is critical not to overwork the batter; it should still be lumpy.
4. Bake for about 15 minutes at 400° in 16 well-greased muffin cups.
5. Remove when the tops are nicely browned and set aside to cool somewhat.

Nutrition: Calories: 154, Proteins: 62 g, Carbs: 40 g, Fat: 5 g

CHAPTER 7:
Snacks

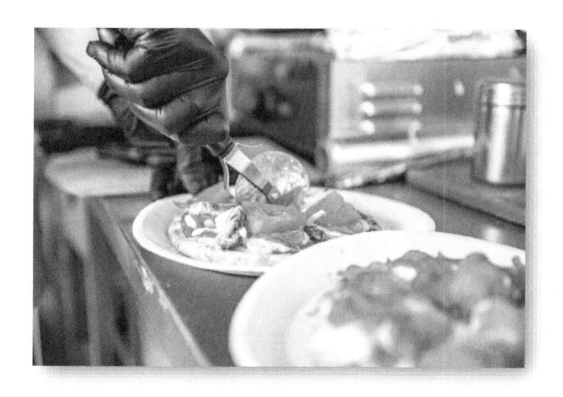

96. Cookie Cup Tarts

Preparation Time: 10 minutes

Cooking Time: 30 minutes

Servings: 3

Ingredients:

- ½ Carton blueberries
- Pre-made sugar cookies
- 2 c. Cool whip
- Mandarin oranges
- 1 kiwi
- 8x10 pan-place cookies

Directions:

1. Make rounds out from either homemade candy cookie dough or bought sugar cookies.
2. Bake the prepared cookie dough in muffin tins for 13 to 15 minutes at 350F.
3. When the cookie cups have cooled, place them on a cake stand or presentation tray.
4. Begin by doling out tablespoons of Cool Whip for the cookie tart's topping. A few teaspoons of Cool Whip should be spread over a cookie cup tart. You can pick whatever color you like!

I like adding color to my cookies by combining mandarin oranges, blueberries, and kiwis with strawberries. It is also an excellent way to include your children in cooking!

Nutrition: Calories: 290, Proteins: 3.4 g, Carbs: 45 g, Fat: 7.1 g

97. Fruit and Ginger Popsicles

Preparation Time: 10 minutes

Cooking Time: 20 minutes

Servings: 2

Ingredients:

- Empty ice cube tray
- Popsicle sticks
- Blender
- 2 tbsps. Greek yogurt
- 2-3 Blueberries
- 1 tsp. Ginger
- 1 slice Mango
- 2 tbsps. Orange juice

Directions:

1. Blend the ingredients until they have a smooth consistency.
2. Insert popsicle sticks into the ice cube pans and place them in the freezer for 20 minutes.

Nutrition: Calories: 61, Proteins: 1.5 g, Carbs: 20 g, Fat: 0.4 g

98. Yogurt Bites

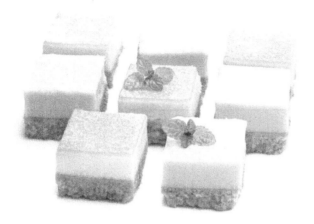

Preparation Time: 5 minutes

Cooking Time: 0 minutes

Servings: 2

Ingredients:

- ½ c. Granola
- ½ c. Raspberries
- 1 small can of Pineapple
- ½ c. Blueberries
- 1 container of vanilla yogurt
- ½ c. Strawberries

Directions:

1. Cover the baking sheet/tray with parchment paper and spread the Greek yogurt evenly. I enjoy creating a variety of cookies so that I may vary the ingredients in different sections of the baking sheet.
2. Level out the yogurt layers with the spatula. Make it thick enough to break apart when it freezes without breaking the whole thing. However, ensure it's flat enough to hold all your toppings.
3. Now comes the exciting part: choose which ingredients to use. Go ahead and make everything similar, with the same components in each element! After it's frozen and hardened, I like to spice it up and separate the components into pieces to choose what I'm most hungry for.
4. On a large baking sheet coated with parchment paper, I divide the fruits, granola, and other items I intend to use. I start with blueberries, crushed pineapple, raspberries, then strawberries. I prefer to add a small range of goods to the remaining sections. On top, I sometimes layer crushed pineapple and blueberries, and other times I layer granola.

5. Place them in the freezer for at least 1 hour after you are satisfied with the layout and toppings.

6. When it is frozen and ready to be broken, cut it into as many or as few pieces as you like. I prefer to place parts in a container easily placed in a refrigerator for an easy snack.

Nutrition: Calories: 564, Proteins: 22.5 g, Carbs: 25 g, Fat: 27.8 g

99. Baked Mushroom Snacks

Preparation Time: 25 minutes

Cooking Time: 16 minutes

Servings: 4

Ingredients:

- 1 clove of garlic, peeled and chopped
- 1 tsp. Salt
- 1 can of mushrooms, plain
- ⅓ tsp. Basil, chopped, fresh, or dried

Directions:

1. Preheat the oven to low and bake the cookie sheet for around ten minutes.
2. Remove the somewhat crispy edges. Take care not to overheat.
3. Put them in a bowl, turn on a movie or favorite show, and enjoy them as a crunchy snack.

Note: Keep a close eye on the snack as they can burn easily in high temperatures.

Nutrition: Calories: 230, Proteins: 35 g, Carbs: 56 g, Fat: 12 g

100. Chili Chickpea

Preparation Time: 5 minutes

Cooking Time: 45 minutes

Servings: 2

Ingredients:

- Garlic powder
- 1 tbsp. Olive oil
- Salt
- Paprika
- 1 ½ tbsp. nutritional yeast
- Onion powder
- 1 15-oz. can chickpeas
- Chili powder

Directions:

1. Preheat the oven to 400°F.
2. Rinse and wash chickpeas thoroughly, making sure they are completely dry.
3. Drizzle with olive oil.
4. Season with nutritional yeast, salt, and pepper to taste, and toss.
5. Preheat the oven to 400°F and bake for 45 minutes, stirring occasionally.

Nutrition: Calories: 98, Proteins: 38 g, Carbs: 90 g, Fat: 7 g

101. Peanut Butter Snack

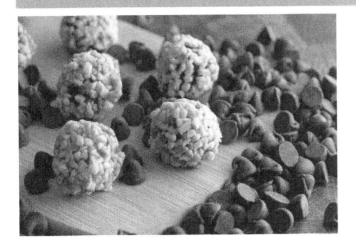

Preparation Time: 10 minutes

Cooking Time: 15 minutes

Servings: 2

Ingredients:

- ½ c. wheat germ
- ½ c. peanut butter
- ½ c. honey
- 1 c. oatmeal

Directions:

1. Combine all ingredients in a mixing bowl.
2. Create 25 "snacks" with a little melon ball-sized tool.

Nutrition: Calories: 150, Proteins: 56 g, Carbs: 30 g, Fat: 6 g

102. Pita Snacks

Preparation Time: 10 minutes

Cooking Time: 15 minutes

Servings: 3

Ingredients:

- 4 pitas (preferably made with almond, coconut, or any ulcerative colitis-friendly flour)
- 8 tbsps. fruit-flavored cream cheese
- Sliced fruits of your choice

Directions:

1. Cut pitas in half to make 8 pockets. Fruit can be sliced or chopped.
2. Fill each pocket with 1 tablespoon of cream cheese.
3. Fill with your favorite pre-cut fruit and enjoy.

Nutrition: Calories: 230, Proteins: 56 g, Carbs: 40 g, Fat: 7 g

103. Cheesy Potato Frittata

Preparation Time: 20 minutes

Cooking Time: 10 minutes

Servings: 2

Ingredients:

- 1 (10 oz.) package of frozen chopped spinach
- 1 c. shredded Daiya Cheddar cheese
- ¼ c. earth balance vegan butter
- 1 c. vegan sour cream
- ¼ tsp. dried dill weed
- Pepper to taste
- 1 tsp. salt
- 6 potatoes, peeled and chopped
- 1 leek, sliced and sauteed

Directions:

1. Preheat the oven to 375°F (175°C).
2. Prepare a medium-sized casserole dish by lightly greasing it. According to the package directions, cook the spinach.
3. Place the potatoes in a large pot with enough water to cover them and come to a boil. Boil for 15 minutes or until soft but still firm. Drain, allow to cool slightly, and then mash.
4. In a small amount of olive oil, sauté the leeks until soft.
5. In a mixing bowl, combine the spinach, leeks, potato salad, vegan butter, sour cream, salt, pepper, and dill.
6. Transfer to the previously prepared casserole dish and top with some Cheddar cheese.
7. Bake for 20 minutes in a preheated oven or until the cheese is bubbling, melted, and golden brown.

Nutrition: Calories: 160, Proteins: 5 g, Carbs: 3 g, Fat: 2 g

104. Haystack Yummy

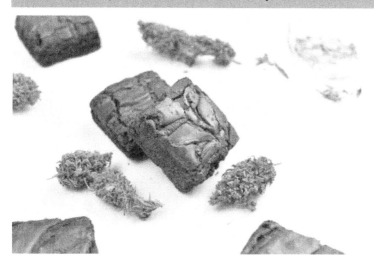

Preparation Time: 10 minutes

Cooking Time: 5 minutes

Servings: 2

Ingredients:

- 1 bag of milk chocolate
- 1 box of fiber
- 1 original brand of cereal
- 24 cupcake liners or wax paper

Directions:

1. Melt an entire bag of Nestle Rippled Milk Chocolate with Peanut Butter Morsels in the microwave.
2. Once the morsels have melted, add half of the Fiber Two Original Label Cereal. Mix until all of the morsels are distributed evenly throughout the cereal.
3. Fill each muffin cup with one or two cupcake papers. Fill 24 cupcake liners evenly with the morsels and Fiber One mixture and chill for 10 minutes to firm up.
4. To avoid melting, keep the haystacks in the fridge in a container.

Nutrition: Calories: 150, Proteins: 26 g, Carbs: 54 g, Fat: 5 g

105. Crispy Rice Snacks

Preparation Time: 20 minutes

Cooking Time: 20 minutes

Servings: 2

Ingredients:

- 5 c. agave
- 5 c. chopped nuts
- 5 c. peanut butter
- 5 tsp. cinnamon
- 5 tsp. vanilla extract
- Erewhon Crispy Brown Rice Cereal

Directions:

1. Mix the peanut oil, agave, nuts, vanilla, and cinnamon in a mixing bowl.
2. Slowly stir in the cereal until it is evenly coated.
3. Use a little cookie scoop to make the balls.
4. Roll the coconut balls in it. Refrigeration may be necessary to preserve the shape.

Nutrition: Calories: 236, Proteins: 75 g, Carbs: 34 g, Fat: 11 g

106. Gluten-Free Trail

Preparation Time: 10 minutes

Cooking Time: 10 minutes

Servings: 5

Ingredients:

- 1 c. Regular or golden raisins, or ½ regular and ½ golden raisins
- 2 c. Dried cranberries
- 1 ½ c. Unsalted peanuts
- ¼ c. Sunflower and pumpkin seeds, raw, shelled

Directions:

1. In a mixing bowl, combine all the fruits and nuts.
2. By dividing 24 portions (into snack baggies), each part will have around 120 calories.

Nutrition: Calories: 140, Proteins: 78 g, Carbs: 70 g, Fat: 9 g

107. Coconut Balls

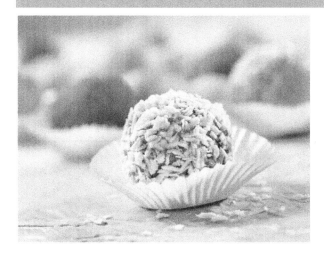

Preparation Time: 30 minutes
Cooking Time: 0 minutes
Servings: 10

Ingredients:

- Almonds
- 2-4 tbsps. virgin coconut oil
- Walnuts
- Pumpkin seeds
- Pecan nuts
- Hazelnuts
- 3-6 dates

Directions:

1. Grind the nuts and pumpkin seeds finely into nut flour using a food processor.
2. Remove the nut flour and blend the dates and chopped coconut in a food processor until smooth.
3. Combine these ingredients with the coffee and chocolate powder to taste.
4. Finally, drizzle in the canola oil and combine everything by hand. Form the paste into tiny balls and roll them in coconut flakes.
5. Refrigerate before serving.

Note: As a starting point, using ½ cup of each nut will yield more than a dozen tiny balls. Dates add richness and help the balls keep their shape, so if the paste isn't holding its shape, add a few more. Coconut oil might also help in this area. Spread the paste equally in a baking tray and top with coconut if you don't have the patience to form a dozen or more little balls. Colting's Cocoa and Cocoa Snacks are a great way to satisfy your midday hunger, whether you eat them as balls or bars.

Nutrition: Calories: 270, Proteins: 78 g, Carbs: 80 g, Fat: 9 g

108. Buffalo Chicken Dip

Preparation Time: 20 minutes

Cooking Time: 20 minutes

Servings: 5

Ingredients:

- 3/8 c. (or 6 tbsps.) Hot sauce (such as Franks')
- ¾ c. Shredded cheddar cheese
- ½ c. Ranch dressing
- 2 cans (5 oz.) of white chicken, drained
- 1 oz. Cream cheese

Directions:

1. Preheat the oven to 350°F.
2. Cook the chicken and spicy sauce over medium heat until well heated. In a mixing dish, combine cream cheese and ranch dressing. Cook, stirring regularly until everything is well mixed and hot.
3. Half of the shredded cheese should be added before transferring the mixture to a 9" x 9" baking sheet. Cover and bake until hot and bubbling, then top with the remaining cheese (about 20 minutes).
4. To serve, toss with tortilla chips.

Nutrition: Calories: 159, Proteins: 79 g, Carbs: 39 g, Fat: 5 g

109. Chocolate Chia Balls

Preparation Time: 15 minutes

Cooking Time: 20 minutes

Servings: 8

Ingredients:

- ½ c. Old Fashioned Oats
- 1 tbsp. Cacao Powder (unsweetened)
- ½ c. Natural Creamy Peanut Butter
- 1 - 1 ½ tbsp. honey
- 1 tbsp. Chia Seeds
- ¼ Dried Cranberries
- 1 scoop of 100-ISO Hydrolyzed Whey Protein Isolate Powder (any flavor)
- 1 Caramel Corn Rice Cake

Directions:

1. In a food processor with a metal blade, combine peanut butter, flax seeds, oats, unsweetened chocolate, 1 tablespoon of honey, and protein.
2. Switch to a mixing or rubber blade and add the dried cranberries, breaking them up and carefully putting them into the food processor.
3. Add another half tablespoon of honey, if necessary, to roll into a ball.
4. To make the balls, measure them with a small cookie scoop and place them on a tray to freeze for about 20 minutes.

Nutrition: Calories: 180, Proteins: 45 g, Carbs: 78 g, Fat: 9 g

110. Super Bowl Snack

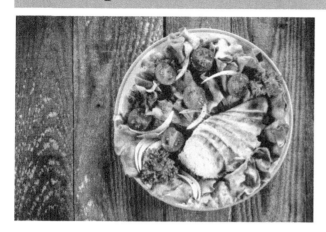

Preparation Time: 10 minutes

Cooking Time: 15 minutes

Servings: 3

Ingredients:

- Slices of low-fat turkey lunchmeat
- 40 grape tomatoes
- 20 baby dill pickles

Directions:

1. Wash and dry tomatoes before cooking. After that, skewer one onto each hors d'oeuvre pick.
2. Remove the pickles from the liquid. To keep it from becoming overly juicy, softly pat it with a paper towel.
3. Cut the turkey stack in half. Wrap a half slice of beef around the pickle, sealing it with two picks, one already bearing the grape tomato. Then, cut the covered pickle in half between the picks.

Nutrition: Calories: 130, Proteins: 67 g, Carbs: 50 g, Fat: 6 g

111. Sweet Potato Hummus

Preparation Time: 15 minutes

Cooking Time: 0 minutes

Servings: 4

Ingredients:

- ½ tsp. garlic
- 1 pinch of cayenne pepper
- 1 4-oz. red peppers
- 15 oz. baked sweet potatoes
- 3 tbsps. Lemon juice
- ½ tsp. ground cumin
- 1 tbsp. Fresh parsley
- ¼ tsp. salt

Directions:

1. In a food processor, combine the sweet potatoes, roasted red peppers, lime juice, garlic, cardamom, cayenne pepper, and salt until smooth.
2. In a food processor, process the ingredients until almost entirely smooth.
3. In the refrigerator, chill the mixture for at least an hour before serving.
4. Sprinkle with the sweet potato and parsley hummus before serving.
5. When there is a flare-up, leave out the cayenne.

Nutrition: Calories: 130, Fat: 0 g, Sodium: 460 mg, Protein: 3 g, Carbs: 28 g

112. Zucchini Chips

Preparation Time: 5 minutes

Cooking Time: 5 minutes

Servings: 2

Ingredients:

- Salt and pepper to taste
- 1 tsp. olive oil
- 1 zucchini medium

Directions:

1. Thinly slice raw zucchini into rounds. Toss the rounds in a bowl with canola oil, salt, and pepper.
2. On a dehydrating sheet, place each round flat and separate. They must not be overlapping as they will not dry properly otherwise.
3. Set the dehydrator to 135°F or 140°F and dry them for 4-5 hours or until crispy.
4. Serve with guacamole, Spanish rice, or hummus. Alternatively, you can eat them plain. In any case, they're fantastic.

Nutrition: Calories: 36, Protein: 1 g, Carbs: 1 g, Fat: 4 g

113. Caramel Energy Bites

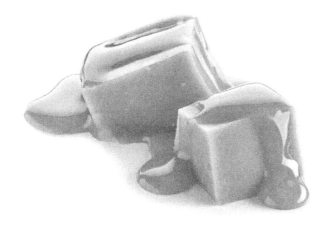

Preparation Time: 40 minutes

Cooking Time: 0 minutes

Servings: 20

Ingredients:

- 1 c. cashew
- 1 c. dates
- ½ tbsp. cinnamon
- 2 tbsps. hemp hearts
- 2 tbsps. cashew butter
- 1 c. coconut
- 2 tbsps. maple syrup

Directions:

1. Combine the dates and cashews in a blender or food processor. Blend the ingredients until it resembles coarse sand.
2. With the coconut, hemp oil, cashew butter, nectar, sea salt, and cinnamon, process until a dough forms.
3. Press the dough between your fingers if it doesn't stick together. Form a one-inch ball with your palms and place it on a parchment-lined dish.
4. Freeze for at least 60 minutes before serving. Freeze them in sealed containers for best results, but they can also be kept in the fridge.

Nutrition: Calories: 103, Protein: 2 g, Carbs: 12 g, Fat: 6 g

114. Coconut Tofu Tenders

Preparation Time: 30 minutes

Cooking Time: 40 minutes

Servings: 4

Ingredients:

- ⅔ c. coconut
- Juice of ½ a lemon
- ½ c. coconut milk
- ¼ tsp. salt
- 2 tbsps. Tahini
- ¼ tsp. pepper
- 1 (14 oz.) firm tofu
- 1 tsp. Hot sauce
- ½ tsp. tamari
- ¼ c. rice cereal

Directions:

1. Preheat the oven to 400°F.
2. On a cutting board, place the tofu and cover it with a clean towel. Set a timer for 20 minutes and place heavy books on the towels.
3. After pressing the tofu, fold it into pieces. Set aside.
4. Mix shredded coconut, cereal, salt, and pepper in a small bowl.
5. Get your "assembly line" set up. Half-fill a small bowl with coconut milk. Dredge the tofu strips in the coconut milk, then transfer them to the coconut-cereal dish to coat. Continue with the remaining strips on a parchment-lined baking sheet.
6. For 20 minutes, bake the tofu strips, flip them over and bake for another 20 minutes.
7. To make the sauce, whisk together all ingredients until a pourable texture is achieved.

Nutrition: Calories: 237, Protein: 10 g, Carbs:13 g, Fat: 17 g

115. Falafel

Preparation Time: 15 minutes

Cooking Time: 10 minutes

Servings: 2

Ingredients:

- 1 garlic clove
- 2 tbsps. almond flour
- ½ onion peeled and chopped
- 400g chickpeas drained and washed
- 1 tbsp. Mango chutney
- 2 tbsps. Olive oil
- 1 tsp. Coriander ground
- 1 tsp. Cumin ground

Directions:

1. Heat 1 tablespoon of oil in a frying pan/saucepan and add the garlic, coriander, onion, and cumin. Cook, occasionally stirring, until the garlic and onions are soft.
2. Puree the chickpeas and flour together in a food processor. Mix in the mango chutney one more time.
3. Roll the mixture into golf-ball-sized beads and flatten them to make about 7-8 falafels. Cook the falafel in the remaining oil for several minutes until golden brown.
4. Serve with extra pita bread, tabbouleh, mango chutney, yogurt, or salad.

Nutrition: Calories: 333, Proteins: 13 g, Carbs: 31.8 g, Fat: 17.8 g

116. Swede Chips

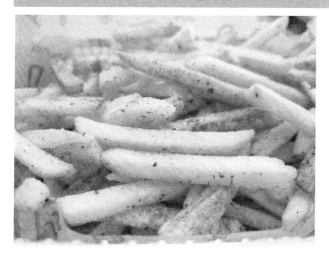

Preparation Time: 10 minutes

Cooking Time: 30 minutes

Servings: 2

Ingredients:

- 2 tbsps. Soy Sauce
- 1 tbsp. Olive Oil
- 1 tbsp. Paprika smoked
- 1 Swede

Directions:

1. Preheat your oven to 200°C.
2. Cut the swede and dice it into chip-sized pieces.
3. Place in a pot of water for 5 minutes before transferring to an oven-safe dish. Mix the swede with olive oil, soy sauce, and paprika to coat.
4. Cook in the oven for about 35 minutes, rotating periodically.

Nutrition: Calories: 52, Proteins: 2 g, Carbs: 10 g, Fat: 0.5 g

117. Spicy Pineapple Salsa

Preparation Time: 20 minutes

Cooking Time: 20 minutes

Servings: 3

Ingredients:

- Hot chili peppers
- 60g onions, raw
- 2 tbsps. Cilantro, raw
- 200g pineapple, fresh
- 100g avocados
- 1 tsp. Packed brown sugar
- 1 tbsp. Fresh mint
- 1 tsp. Olive oil
- Juice from 1 lime
- 5g of ginger root

Directions:

1. Boil potatoes in a pot and allow them to cool after boiling.
2. Boil the eggs in boiling water and allow them to boil slowly or simmer for 7 minutes. Place the eggs in a dish with ice water to lower their temperature.
3. While the potatoes and eggs cook, dice the pickles and set them aside. After the eggs and potatoes have cooled, cube them and combine them with the diced pickles and onions in a big mixing bowl.
4. Mash the egg yolks; you don't have to use them all.
5. Combine the mayonnaise, mustard, and sweet relish in the same bowl; add enough dill cucumber juice to soften the mayonnaise and mustard, and season to taste.

Nutrition: Calories: 200, Proteins: 50 g, Carbs: 20 g, Fat: 9 g

118. Angel Pasta

Preparation Time: 35 minutes

Cooking Time: 25 minutes

Servings: 4

Ingredients:

- Large cloves of garlic, thinly sliced
- 2 tsp. Grated lemon zest
- 1 ½ tbsp. Extra-virgin olive oil
- ¼ tsp. crushed red pepper
- 2 oz. large peeled, deveined raw shrimp
- Unsalted butter, cut into pieces
- ¾ c. finely chopped yellow onion
- 2 oz. white angel hair pasta
- 2 tbsps. Lemon juice
- ¼ tsp. salt
- 2 tbsps. dry white wine
- ⅓ c. grated Parmesan cheese
- ¼ c. chopped parsley

Directions:

1. Prepare pasta "al dente" by boiling it in a large saucepan according to the package directions.
2. Drain, reserving half a cup of the cooking liquid. Place aside.
3. In a large saucepan over medium heat, heat the oil. Cook the onion, garlic, and lemon zest over medium heat, stirring regularly, for about 5 minutes or until the onion is soft.
4. Add the shrimp and crushed red pepper. Turn and flip the shrimp regularly, for about 3 minutes, or until the shrimp are just a touch translucent in the center.
5. Add the wine and cook for another 30 seconds while stirring. After rinsing the pasta, add the butter, residual boiling water, and a half-cup. Raise the heat and cook the sauce, constantly stirring with tongs, for 1 to 2 minutes or until it achieves a creamy consistency.
6. While stirring, add the parsley, lemon juice, and salt.
7. Divide evenly among 4 bowls and garnish with more chopped parsley if desired.

Nutrition: Calories: 300, Proteins: 60 g, Carbs: 60 g, Fat: 23 g

119. Nice Cream Sundae

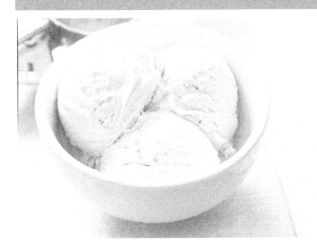

Preparation Time: 30 minutes

Cooking Time: 0 minutes

Servings: 2

Ingredients:

- 4 ripe bananas
- ½ c. oat milk/almond milk
- ½ tsp. vanilla extract

Directions:

1. Add frozen banana slices, milk, and vanilla essence to a blender and blend until smooth.
2. Place in the bowl and garnish with chosen toppings.
3. Serve instantly and enjoy.

Nutrition: Calories: 112, Proteins: 1.4 g, Carbs: 27.3 g, Fat: 0.8 g

120. Garden Frittata

Preparation Time: 5 minutes

Cooking Time: 25 minutes

Servings: 3

Ingredients:

- 4 large organic eggs
- ½ tsp. salt
- ½ bell pepper
- 1 medium tomato
- 1 tbsp. fresh chives
- ½ c. cheese

Directions:

1. Preheat your oven to 400°F and prepare a large skillet with frying spray. Set to the side.
2. Whisk the eggs and salt in a large bowl, then add chopped veggies, chives, and goat cheese. Whisk to mix the ingredients.
3. Pour the mixture into the pan, then top with the remaining goat cheese.
4. Bake for 15 minutes. Remove from heat and cool for 5 minutes before serving.

Nutrition: Calories: 83, Proteins: 6.5 g, Carbs: 3 g, Fat: 5.6 g

CHAPTER 8:
28 Days Meal Plan

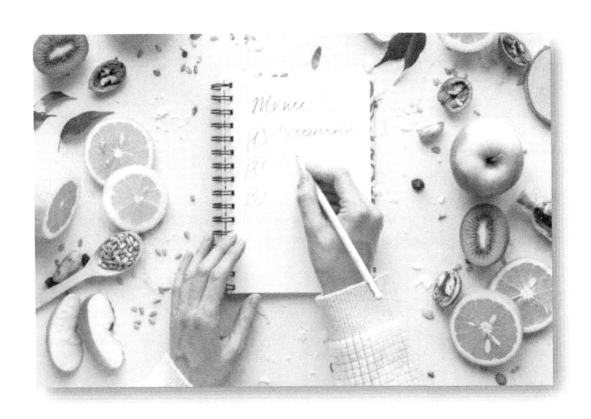

Day	Breakfast	Lunch	Dinner	Dessert
1	Bacon, Avocado, And Eggs	Ground Chicken With Tomatoes	Cantaloupe Gnocchi	Vegan Granola Cups
2	Breakfast Berry Crisp	Egg and Avocado Endive Wraps	Rosemary Chicken	Tofu Chocolate Cake
3	Golden Overnight Oats With Orange Flavor	Pasta With Asparagus	Winter Apple Poke Bowl	Free Dairy Banana Chocolate Ice Cream
4	Mediterranean Eggplant Shakshuka	Beef and Mozzarella Burgers	Shrimp Salmon Tomato Stew	Java Bananas
5	Avocado-Egg Salad Toast	Lemony Scallops	Shrimp Scampi Pizza	Free Gluten And Dairy Apple Crumb
6	Muffins With Morning Glory	Shrimp Lettuce Wraps	Turkey With Rosemary	Fried Honey Bananas
7	Bacon-Wrapped Chicken, Pineapple, Roasted Veggies	Turkey Burgers	Zero-Fiber Chicken Dish	Eggless Honey Cake
8	Soup Of Butternut Squash	Beef and Veggie Burgers	Chicken Cacciatore	Blueberry Galette
9	Apple And Banana Pancakes	Liver With Onion And Parsley	Whole Roasted Trout	Mocha Ricotta Crème
10	Chocolate Zucchini Muffins	Beef and Spinach Burgers	Lemon Pepper Turkey	Banana Cupcakes
11	Frittatas With Spinach And Red Peppers	Pasta With Zucchini and Tomatoes	Stuffed Zucchini Boats	Orange Muffins

12	Green Peanut Butter-Banana Smoothie	Roasted Pumpkin Curry	Lemony Salmon	Free Dairy Chocolate Hazelnut Spread
13	Sweet Potato, Egg, And Avocado Breakfast	Chicken Lettuce Wraps	Prawn and Tomato Spaghetti	Autumnal Vegan Carrots With Walnuts
14	Egg, Turkey, And Cheese Breakfast Sandwich	Pan-Seared Scallops	Grilled Salmon Steaks	Christmas In A Cup
15	Sweet Potato Ginger Pancakes	Shrimp Tomato Salad	Fiesta Chicken Tacos	Royal Crown Pie
16	Lemon Bars	Beef Skewers	Duck With Pear	Custard Dairy Free
17	Smoked Salmon Frittata	Versatile Mac 'N Cheese	Brazilian Fish Stew	Vegan Pecan Tart With Chocolate Crust
18	Blueberry Pancakes With Oatmeal	Tuna Stuffed Avocado	Turkey And Kale Sauté	Gluten- And Dairy-Free Blueberry Cupcakes With Lemon Icing
19	Orange And Honey Duck	Shrimp and Tomato Bake	Chicken Cutlets	Dairy- And Gluten-Free Carrot Cake
20	Gingerbread Waffles	European Beet Soup	Halibut Curry	Pink Lemonade Pie
21	Egg Bake	Potatoes With Tomatoes	Herbed Salmon	Sweet Dessert Bliss
22	Green Peanut Butter-Banana Smoothie	Tomato Salmon Bowl	Veggie Risotto	Brownie Bites

23	Sweet Potato, Egg, And Avocado Breakfast	Greek Cucumber Salad	Chicken Piccata	Flourless Cake
24	Egg, Turkey, And Cheese Breakfast Sandwich	Fried Rice With Kale	Easiest Tuna Salad	Avocado Sorbet
25	Bacon, Avocado, And Eggs	Beef and Spinach Burgers	Peach Stew	Banana Cupcakes
26	Avocado-Egg Salad Toast	Pasta With Zucchini and Tomatoes	Chicken Cacciatore	Orange Muffins
27	Muffins With Morning Glory	Roasted Pumpkin Curry	Whole Roasted Trout	Free Dairy Chocolate Hazelnut Spread
28	Bacon-Wrapped Chicken, Pineapple, Roasted Veggies	Chicken Lettuce Wraps	Lemon Pepper Turkey	Autumnal Vegan Carrots With Walnuts

CHAPTER 9:
FAQ

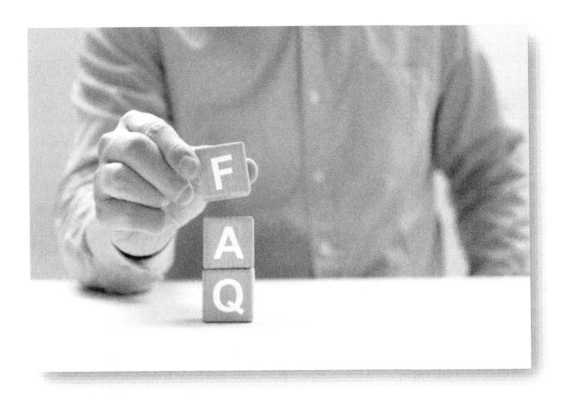

1. **What causes ulcerative colitis?**

Researchers believe that the causes of ulcerative colitis are numerous and complex. They attribute this to an overactive immune response. The immune system defends the body against viruses and other potentially harmful components. However, your immune system can accidentally attack your body, causing tissue damage and swelling.

2. **If you have ulcerative colitis, what foods are you allowed to eat?**

There is no single diet that will miraculously cure ulcerative colitis. During remission, your diet will most likely differ from that of disease flares. It is vital to consume a nutrient-rich diet when in remission to keep healthy.

- Fiber-rich Foods: These include beans, barley, almonds, oat bran, and whole grains. A low-fiber diet is advised if you have an ostomy, intestinal restriction, or have recently had surgery.
- High-Protein Dietary Sources: These include poultry, fish, eggs, and tofu.
- Vegetables and Fruits: Eating all the vegetables and fruits you can think of is important. No matter what, as long as they are fruits and vegetables, they are good for you.
- Calcium-Rich Foods: Some calcium-rich foods include yogurt, milk (if you are not lactose-intolerant), and collard greens.

3. What foods should you eat when you have a flare?

According to the Crohn's and Colitis Foundation, consuming bland, easily digestible foods is often beneficial during a flare-up.

4. What sets off a flare-up?

The short answer is that doctors don't know what causes IBD in the first place, and flares can happen at any time during the disease. Sometimes the large intestine muscles do not contract or stretch adequately to aid in food digestion, or the patient has difficulties breaking down food due to an overly sensitive gut prone to generating gas and bloating, a condition known as "Leaky Gut Syndrome." Current medical studies are looking into the biological impact of sleep and exercise on IBD symptoms and general health. Many of us know that stress has a long-term and considerable impact on all diseases. Stress and the hormones released during stressful events directly impact our health. Our way of life greatly impacts the prevalence of many diseases, including IBD.

5. When is it best to go see a doctor?

Even though ulcerative colitis seldom leads to death, it is a serious condition with potentially fatal effects. If you have ulcerative colitis symptoms but have not yet been diagnosed, you should immediately see a doctor. They can examine samples of your blood or stool to see what is causing your symptoms. If additional tests are required, you may be admitted to the hospital.

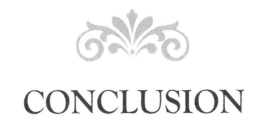

CONCLUSION

Thank you for reading this book. Every patient suffering from ulcerative colitis must actively participate in their treatment. They should be aware of the depth of their disease, the treatments they've taken, what has and hasn't helped, and whether or not they've had any adverse effects and what those consequences were. Because Ulcerative Colitis is a chronic condition that will affect you for the rest of your life, you should choose the correct healthcare provider to assist you in effectively managing your illness.

You should notify your doctor if your current treatment does not yield satisfactory results. You and your healthcare provider can collaborate to develop the best diet plan and medication treatment for your Ulcerative Colitis condition.

Keeping a food journal will help you determine which foods cause your symptoms. This is also significant since you will know how to avoid a flare-up by not eating or drinking anything that produces symptoms. With a food journal, you can eat various foods and record which foods cause a flare-up. Doing this will help you make better food choices. Even the best meals might aggravate symptoms, so keeping track of your "problem foods" may be beneficial. Any inquiries about healthy eating should be referred to your healthcare physician.

One of the most important things you can do for yourself if you have Ulcerative Colitis is to be your own advocate. When discussing with your doctors, do not be scared to express yourself. Ask as many questions as you want, and be open about your feelings about the treatment you're receiving.

Ulcerative Colitis can be hard on your stomach, and you may need to change your diet during a flare-up, possibly sticking to a BRAT diet of banana, rice, applesauce, and toast. So, if you achieve remission, you may be able to celebrate by eating foods that make you happy while also tasting delicious. However, you should proceed with caution to avoid accidentally worsening your symptoms.

You can eat more small meals instead of three large ones, especially if you're on the road or don't have convenient access to a restroom. Eat foods you know will help you manage your symptoms if you've just had a flare-up. You can prepare meals you can eat both at home and work beforehand. If you plan to go on a trip, consult your family doctor, who can advise you on what to do if you get a flare-up while driving or traveling. You will feel much better and be able to manage your symptoms as a result of this. Living with ulcerative colitis can be extremely difficult, so learning about it and how to manage it is vital.

Good luck!

Made in United States
North Haven, CT
15 April 2023

35477784R00089